OVERCOME AUTOIMMUNE DISEASE

An instructive guide on autoimmune conditions like lupus, rheumatoid arthritis, Hashimoto's Thyroiditis – and more – and what you can do to manage or reverse them.

2024
ECOLOGICAL NUTRITION
Ballarat, Victoria

For everyone out there struggling with an autoimmune disease – a better life is out there, waiting for you. You've already taken the first step towards it.

Table of Contents

3

Disclaimer

Though prepared by a certified health professional, the following information is general and, therefore, should not be treated as medical advice.

Prelude

The Most Important Thing I Did to Heal from Autoimmune Disease Was Believe

"Whether you think you can or you can't – you're right."

Henry Ford

To all outward appearances, I was vital and healthy when I was 30. But behind the scenes, I had all sorts of health issues.

I knew some of what I was grappling with; I dealt with it daily.

Yet, at the same time, I was in denial. If you'd asked me, I'd have said my health was perfect. The asthma that I had as a child was gone. I was conscientious about my diet and exercised most days. I had no issues with weight. I had a bachelor's degree with first-class honours (honours is a mini-PhD we do in Australia).

I was also running an acclaimed small business and touted as someone shaping the future of my industry. The picture-perfect success story.

But the harsh reality was I was far from healthy. I suffered from a severe sleep deficiency. I yo-yoed between anxiety and depression for years. Then, I developed symptoms of complex post-traumatic stress disorder (CPTSD) alongside mysterious physical complaints. Despite running numerous tests, the doctor I saw couldn't find a cause for them.

The Downward Spiral

One of my most prominent symptoms was fatigue. I felt exhausted. When I got home from work, I'd collapse on the floor in front of the bar heater I'd bought for my small apartment and drift off to sleep. My cat would wake me up in the early morning hours, bewildered that I wasn't in bed. One night, I fell into such a deep sleep that there were burns on my hands and arms from being too close to the heater when I awoke at 2 am.

Panic attacks were a regular feature in my day, sometimes many times. Sometimes, specific events triggered them. Other times, I was simply overwhelmed by my racing thoughts.

Disconnected from the people around me, I lived in my own personal hell. It was a lonely place to be: if I didn't fall asleep in front of the heater, I would often cry myself to sleep.

Despite eating less and being active, I started gaining weight. When I was 15, I had developed anorexia. My obsession with caloric restriction and thinness lasted several years, so I knew all the tricks to lose weight. It was disconcerting to discover that none of them worked anymore.

Concentration became an issue. I had to write things down immediately or risk forgetting them. Once-simple cognitive tasks became a struggle. Business management and future planning were beyond more. Simply focusing on the here and now was challenging.

At the end of 2017, I decided to close my business. This was a heart-wrenching decision. After an employee spectacularly blew their budget, the business' financial struggles were adding to the mountain of stress I was already dealing with. I had a sense that if I didn't shut it down, I would not make it through whatever was going on. I had lost all joy in life. It was time for a change.

Yet closing the business caused additional stress. There were suppliers, many of them friends, to whom the business owed money. I felt terrible, blaming myself for everything that went wrong.

And the more guilt and shame I felt, the more my symptoms continued to worsen. My hair, always so thick and healthy, began falling out in clumps. My hormones were already a mess: I was lucky if I had my cycle four or five times a year. My muscles shrank, taking my strength with them. Every morning became a delicate dance with my limbs' worsening aches and pains. My joints hurt as well, rendering movement a struggle. Exercise and rigorous movement made things worse. Only gentle stretching helped.

Meanwhile, I received threatening text messages, phone calls, and emails from a handful of business creditors. After a car followed me home from an evening walk in the park, I also suspected that an ex was stalking me. Soon after, a neighbour left a note about someone hanging around outside my bathroom window.

Nightmares replaced my dreams. Thoughts of what could happen next terrified me. I'm small and female, with no knowledge of self-defence. I'm sure you can imagine some of the scenes that played out in my mind and woke me up in a cold sweat at night.

Following the business closure, I moved to rural New South Wales (NSW) and lived with my uncle's family, desperate for time out of the city. Submersing myself in the warm embrace of family gave me some reprieve from stress.

But I knew that it was a temporary move; I wouldn't be staying forever. I didn't have a job or any prospects there. Nevertheless, I stayed for the better part of a year, taking each day slowly.

Even though I didn't look particularly unwell, my health was so poor that I was barely functional. Most days, simply getting out of bed was a struggle.

On the nights when nightmares didn't plague my sleep, I dreamed of the ocean right near where I grew up. I dreamed of the cool, aquamarine water on my skin, the squeaky sand beneath my feet, the sea breeze in my hair, and the sun's warm rays.

One morning, after waking from one such dream, I knew what my subconscious had been trying to tell me. What I needed most. In late 2018, I moved back to my childhood home. A cattle farm near Esperance on the southeast coast of Western Australia with my parents.

There was an incredible sense of relief when I arrived there. After six months, my symptoms abated to the point where I started to feel I had a future again. Things still weren't right, but I felt hopeful of regaining control of my health and my life.

Getting a Diagnosis

At the start of 2020, I was feeling well enough to start my PhD at the University of Western Australia. I had no taste for an academic career but was sure I could do it and felt the need to challenge myself again. I also felt my wine industry experience and project on adopting regenerative agriculture could, too.

I moved to Perth as COVID-19 hit, with the city going into lockdown the weekend I moved. I had plenty of time on my hands to conduct research, not only for my PhD but also for my ongoing health condition. I suspected I had Hashimoto's Thyroiditis, even though it hadn't shown up on the testing that I'd done for it back in 2017. But as I began to read more about it, I realised that I hadn't had the right testing done.

I went to another doctor and requested a complete thyroid panel. The doctor refused. She would only test my thyroid stimulating hormone (TSH) and tetraiodothyronine (T4). These are standard tests for suspected thyroid issues but my research suggested they might be normal, even if my thyroid was the issue.

That doctor wasn't available the day my results came back and I was so keen to get them that I booked in with another doctor from the same clinic. Again, nothing showed up. He even went so far as to tell me was too thin to have Hashimoto's without asking about my diet, exercise, or my weight before I noticed symptoms. He even suggested that I try doing some more exercise if I wanted to lose weight.

By this point, I was determined to uncover the root of my health issues. I decided to get a full thyroid panel done myself. Money was tight, so it seemed like a huge investment at the time. But it was the best $130 I've ever spent because, lo and behold, there were the results I'd been searching for. I finally had a diagnosis of Hashimoto's thyroiditis.

I saw yet another doctor, recommended by a friend, with these new results. She gave me my official diagnosis. For most people, getting a diagnosis of Hashimoto's thyroiditis means going on a medication called levothyroxine. This is an artificial form of thyroid hormone that can help improve metabolism and energy levels. I longed for the relief I knew it would bring. At the same time, I feared its side effects and long-term dependence. In the end, I decided not to take it. I had improved a bit over the last few years. If I could manage it on my own, I would be able to avoid unwanted side effects plus the ongoing expense. She didn't give me any hope of healing, though, stating that I would always need to manage my condition.

She also ordered an ultrasound of my thyroid. It showed micro-nodules, or scarring, from the antibody attacks. This worried me. My research suggested they could become cancerous if not monitored. Everything I read suggested they might not heal without medication, if at all.

Yet, the more I researched, the less true much of what I'd read by experts appeared to be. I had already come a long way on my own, even without knowing what I had. I knew I had a long way to go to be healthy. But this got me wondering: *did it have to be a lifelong condition?*

A few days after my diagnosis, I read a research article on autoimmune diseases. It used the term "epigenetic." A light bulb went off in my head.

If a condition is epigenetic, it means that there is high malleability in the expression of the genes involved.

Epigenetics is a field that studies how genes are expressed. Even though your genes provide a template for who you are, not all of them express themselves at the same time. Genes are a bit like a light in your home; they are always connected to the grid, but whether or not they illuminate a room is dependent on whether you've flicked the switch on or off. Our body has a clever system for turning them on and off at various times, which allows us to be responsive to what's going on around us.

Some of them stay turned on for the rest of your life once they've been activated. Things like eye colour, height, and skin colour tend to be more fixed. However, the article I came across suggested that genes involved in the immune system are more flexible. They're *meant* to turn on and off in response to environmental and physiological cues.

This suggested to me that my autoimmune condition could be temporary. If the genes could be turned on by environmental and physiological cues, environmental and physiological cues might also be able to turn them off.

I became determined to see what I was capable of. While reading this article, I decided to turn off the genes that caused my autoimmune condition. I committed to do everything in my power to do so.

I spent the next few years researching Hashimoto's, implementing what I learned along the way. Every six months, I would go to my doctor for blood tests, and then once a year, she would get my ultrasounds done. I asked her to share the results. I wanted to track my progress, not rely on her view. As we monitored, the numbers underwent a steady shift. My antibodies went down, and all my thyroid hormones improved. My micro-nodules started to heal and fade. During my last ultrasound, the radiologist was unsure about what to look for.

February 2023 marked my official remission confirmation. I had done what doctors and experts had said wasn't possible.

I took no medications. Yet, I was symptom-free, and all the tests showed I had a complete remission of Hashimoto's thyroiditis.

Delving Deeper into Epigenetics

Over the next year, though, something still seemed a little off. I hadn't lost all the extra weight I gained when I was at my worst, so I suspected my metabolism was still a little sluggish. There was another piece of the puzzle missing. I felt as though my health wasn't quite optimal.

Later that year, I began to study genetics and epigenetics after listening to a podcast that mentioned mutations in the methylenetetrahydrofolate reductase (MTHFR) gene. We're going to go into all of this in more detail in an upcoming chapter on genetics, but here's a quick overview of what I learnt.

The MTHFR gene produces a protein that plays a role in methylation, a key process in epigenetic gene expression. A mutation is a change in the DNA sequence that can alter how genes work and sometimes affect traits or health. Mutations in this gene can impair methylation if not fully supported nutritionally. The result is that gene expression is less flexible and responsive than it should be.

If we go back to the light switch analogy of how epigenetics works, this results in the switch not being turned on or off correctly in response to the environment. It's as if someone glued the switch into one position. The light would be perpetually on or off. Either could be problematic. If you wanted to read at night but the light wasn't on, you wouldn't be able to. If you want to get a good sleep, the bright light might keep you awake.

The podcast guest said that mutations in this gene raise the risk of several health issues, including autoimmune diseases.

After more research, I was sure I had the variant in the MTHFR gene that causes the most problems with genetic flexibility. I had had several issues that are commonly associated with it: allergies, anxiety and depression, Hashimoto's, problems with concentration, and more.

Curious, I decided to get my genes tested. Sure enough, there it was. I have two copies of the gene MTHFR 677C>T (the most problematic mutation). In fact, I have many mutations that affect methylation, predisposing me to developing chronic health conditions.

I grasped the immense power of this new knowledge instantly. I could change my diet and lifestyle to target my genes. This might prevent further major health issues, including a relapse.

Putting My Health to the Ultimate Test

Within weeks of changing my diet and supplements to better support my MTHFR gene and methylation more generally, I saw some small but important changes. I had more energy. My metabolism seemed faster. My head felt clearer. I could sit and focus on tasks for hours.

I felt so good that I decided to run a marathon.

Fear gripped me even just thinking about it. Running had been my favourite form of movement pre-Hashimoto's, something that I'd done off and on for years. I'd always wanted to run a marathon, but the timing had never been quite right. I always postponed it for later.

When I could no longer run because of my autoimmune condition, I felt I had lost a part of my identity. It wasn't just that I knew how bad it could be for me. In 2018, when my autoimmune disease had been at its worst, running just a short distance could put me into flares that lasted for days, sometimes weeks. Other times when I had challenged myself too much physically with winemaking, it had come with a heavy cost, taking months to recover.

I needed to overcome two fears to start running again. I feared not being as fast as before. I also feared making myself sick again.

But then I thought back to the many things I'd read when I was first diagnosed with Hashimoto's that said autoimmune diseases aren't curable and that I would need to be on medication. The evidence had shown me something to the contrary. Because I believed what I'd read, I believed in myself and achieved the so-called impossible. Now, my blood tests and ultrasounds showed that I was fully recovered. There was no real reason why I would get sick from it, so long as I took care of myself while I was training and during the actual event.

I'm still not as fast as I was back in my heyday, but in late April 2024, I attempted my first-ever marathon. I finished the first half in one hour and 48 minutes flat. That was an okay time.

The second half was vicious. By around the 30 km mark, my feet were hurting, and pain was shooting up the outside of my thigh from my knee. My shoulders were feeling cramped, and every muscle in my body was screaming at me to stop. I knew I was going to hurt later.

I ran the Ballarat marathon in just over 4 hours and 2 minutes. I was hoping for a little faster, but I'm still so proud of myself for doing it at all! This was a new personal best for me. I felt proud of myself no matter which way I looked at it.

The Most Important Thing is to Believe

I was so exhausted and stiff that my partner had to support me to get into the car when I finished the marathon. Then, he had to carry me inside and into a salt bath. I stayed in there for 40 minutes, trying to loosen up my muscles. It took days to recover enough to walk without pain.

But you know what? Every single bit of pain was worth the feeling I got afterwards. The sense of confidence in myself and my body is without price. I know now that I am capable of far more than I ever gave myself credit for. I didn't only heal myself from an autoimmune disease. I also did something no one would have thought I could do six years ago when my health was at its worst. According to most doctors and the academic literature, I am a medical miracle.

I think it's important that you know I don't have some special gene that makes me a good runner, nor did I have good preparation going in. I strained a groin muscle eight weeks out, so I didn't train much in the two months leading up. I had only been training for two months before that. So, my preparation was decidedly poor. And I had never done a distance greater than a half marathon at that point.

What I did have was determination and belief in myself. I knew deep inside that if I kept on putting one foot in front of the other, I would get to the finish line eventually. I had to slow down to do it, but I got there.

That was my first marathon, but I don't intend for it to be my last. There are more coming up on my horizon. And I want you to know that, however sick you are right now, you too can have a life after autoimmune disease.

The most important thing to overcoming any obstacle, including an autoimmune disease, is committing to do it. If you believe in yourself and apply what you learn in this book, the health that you yearn for will be more than just a dream.

Introduction

"The physician knows that his little black bag can only carry him so far and that the body's own healing system is the main resource."

Norman Cousins

I'm guessing you're reading this because you, or someone close to you, has an autoimmune disease, confirmed or suspected. You may never have heard of autoimmune diseases before now, so you've come to this book to understand the possible causes of your symptoms. Perhaps someone you care about has an autoimmune disease, and you're here to learn.

Whatever the reason, know you and your loved ones are not alone. Autoimmune diseases are rising globally. Some experts are now calling them an epidemic.

A recent study estimated the incidence (new cases) of autoimmune disease to be around 19.1% each year. Meanwhile, the prevalence is increasing by around 12.5% annually (1). Though some people with autoimmune diseases are dying each year and others are going into remission, new diagnoses far outstrip rates of remission and death. The prevalence of autoimmune disease is increasing at an alarming rate.

In the last several years, the awareness of autoimmune conditions seems to have been increasing. There are Facebook groups, online forums, and webinars where people can seek and find answers about them. This partly accounts for their increasing prevalence: more awareness leads to better diagnosis.

But their rate of increase is so rapid that this is only *part* of the picture. It's far more likely that something else is causing their increased prevalence. While genes play a role in the onset and progression of autoimmune diseases, environmental factors account for, on average, 70% of autoimmune disease risk (2). My research and experience in reversing Hashimoto's has taught me that these are lifestyle diseases.

Despite the evidence supporting this conclusion, they're rarely treated as such. I never received any lifestyle counselling or advice from my doctors other than to reduce stress. Though this is an excellent piece of advice, how to go about this or get support was never discussed. Nor were my diet, activity levels, environmental toxin exposures, or sleep discussed.

I hear the same thing from clients with autoimmune diseases: they're rarely informed about just how much control they can have over their health. The status quo is to prescribe medications that, as research shows, do little to address the underlying issues that cause autoimmune diseases. In addition, they can have serious side effects.

Current Diagnoses and Treatments for Autoimmune Diseases Are Failing

Autoimmune diseases—and the symptoms associated with them—are inflammatory conditions. Inflammation is a vital immune response. It's the result of the immune system's strategy to attack harmful pathogens or foreign materials that have breached the body's defences. Its function is to go to war against pathogens. The immune system's inflammatory molecules are its ammo. They seek and destroy pathogens. At the same time, the body sends resources to the immune system. This helps heal damage from the invaders.

So, when and why does inflammation develop into an autoimmune disease?

Chronic, acute inflammation can lead to autoimmune diseases when the immune system malfunctions and becomes so hyper-vigilant that it produces antibodies that attack the self. This causes internal damage to target organs and tissues and those caught in the crossfire. Many symptoms commonly experienced in autoimmune conditions, such as photosensitivity, rashes, and food intolerances, are the consequence of this (3).

Additionally, the immune system uses a lot of energy. As a result, people with autoimmune diseases often feel exhausted. And because it's a systemic response, inflammation causes widespread aches and pains. They're rarely limited to one area of the body. Those with autoimmune disease are often crippled by their condition.

Common treatments for autoimmune disease include anti-inflammatory medications, replacement of organ functions, such as insulin in Type 1 diabetes, immunosuppressing drugs, and immunoglobulin therapy (4).

All have harmful side effects as they may disrupt the health of other organs and systems within your body (5; 6). For example, prednisone, a synthetic corticosteroid commonly used to treat autoimmune diseases, works by suppressing the immune system. But in doing that, it can lead to increased cancer risk and mental health issues (7; 8). Even insulin, which can be life-saving for those with Type 1 Diabetes, comes with risks (9).

In addition, these medications aren't treating the underlying cause of autoimmune diseases. They treat the symptoms. Even though you may not get the same aches and pains as before their use, subclinical disease progression may still take place (10). Further complications like organ damage or secondary health conditions aren't uncommon in autoimmune diseases (11).

My personal experience with Hashimoto's thyroiditis — both diagnosis and treatment — has led me to believe that Western medicine is letting a lot of us down. I know I'm not the only one who feels like this. Many of my clients and people that I know socially with an autoimmune diagnosis feel their doctor isn't listening.

In addition, they feel as though their health and concerns aren't a priority. This was exactly how I felt when a doctor told me I was "too thin" to have Hashimoto's and that I should do more exercise if I wanted to lose some weight. This was in response to me asking him to do more extensive testing to get a diagnosis. I had been ill and incapacitated for three and a half years at that point and experienced a wide range of symptoms indicating autoimmune thyroid disease, yet he didn't seem to care about any of that.

I ordered the tests myself directly after this appointment, so I finally had answers about my health issues within a matter of days. But it would have been easy to get discouraged by his response. Perhaps if I wasn't so stubborn, I would still be waiting on a diagnosis four and a half years later.

Why Are Autoimmune Diseases So Poorly Diagnosed and Treated?

People with autoimmune diseases have reasons to feel fobbed off. I count myself lucky to have received a diagnosis within three and a half years of noticing a significant deterioration in my health. The Autoimmune Association says it takes the average person *seven years* and *five doctors* to get an autoimmune diagnosis in the United States (12). The system doesn't cater to those with autoimmune diseases.

There are a couple of reasons for this.

Autoimmune diseases are complex, so their symptoms overlap with other conditions. Because symptoms like pain and fatigue are subjective, they can be invisible (13). The doctor who refused my request for more extensive testing told me I seemed "fine", yet I was struggling. I knew that every day shouldn't feel so hard. This had me seething inside, but I also felt hurt and alone. No one else knows what your internal experience of wellness or illness feels like. Perhaps understandably, this can make diagnosis complicated, but it's no excuse for doctors not listening to their patients.

In addition, there are no definitive tests for some autoimmune diseases. Diagnoses can be the result of a patchwork of testing that leads to a common aetiology. This adds to diagnostic complexity, and primary care providers often aren't taught how to do everything needed to come to a conclusion (14; 15). No wonder so many patients feel frustrated.

Australian doctors are also discouraged from "overusing" the publicly funded healthcare system for diagnostic testing. Dr Nick Coatsworth says this leads to high-cost, "low-value care" (16). It might save the government money in the short term, but it costs patients — and society — more in the long term. Dr. Lawrence Afrin laments the same issue in America, though in this context, attributable to barriers put in place by insurance companies for the diagnosis of mast cell activation syndrome (MCAS), a condition that underpins autoimmune diseases (17).

Nor is a standard 15-minute (or sometimes shorter!) appointment long enough to go through all of the details surrounding chronic health conditions — let alone their cause (18). It takes me an hour and a half to conduct my first session with a client with an autoimmune disease or any other chronic health issue. Even then, more relevant information will often come out in subsequent appointments.

Additionally, it's worth noting that medicine is more than just a profession. It's an *industry*. Companies make money out of you being sick and stuck on medication for life. In the US alone, it's reported that over $100 billion US dollars is spent on autoimmune disease treatment each year, though this is likely a "gross underestimate" (1). Yet, despite all the claims that pharmaceuticals are the only way to treat autoimmune diseases, the reality is that they're not very effective. We know this is because the number needed to treat (NNT) for most of them is so high.

The NNT is the number of patients that need to be treated before one patient benefits. For example, if a medication has an NNT of 7, seven people need to receive the treatment for one person to experience a benefit that they would not have experienced without the treatment. In other words, for every seven patients treated, one person benefits from the treatment in a way that is attributable to the medication, while the others would either see no benefit or achieve the same outcome without the treatment.

The lower the NNT, the more effective the treatment is. The higher it is, the less effective it is (19).

What do you think the NNT is for medications commonly prescribed in autoimmune diseases?

For methotrexate, used in Rheumatoid Arthritis, it's 4-6 for a 20% reduction in symptoms (20). That's not a cure. It's a one in 5 chance that it might make you a little less tired and achy.

Disease-modifying therapies commonly used in multiple sclerosis, such as interferon-beta or glatirmar acetate, have an NNT of 7–10 to prevent one additional relapse or clinical exacerbation that would have otherwise occurred without the treatment. If you achieve symptom reduction and all you do is one of these therapies, you're more than likely to relapse (21). In addition, they may have limited effects on the neurodegenerative aspects of the disease (22).

And though biologics, some of the most effective of any of the autoimmune medications, often have an NNT of 2 or less for a 75% reduction in symptoms within a few months, they come at a cost (23). The risk of bacterial, fungal, and virus infections is increased due to their immune-suppressing effects (24). Long-term users are also potentially at higher cancer risk (25). Paradoxically, some people may also develop an autoimmune response to biologics, reducing their effectiveness and leading to more medications being added (26). They're also expensive, often priced at thousands of dollars per month (27). You either need to be living somewhere with a well-funded medical system or have comprehensive medical insurance to access them.

Just before this book went to print, I asked people on some online platforms for autoimmune diseases if they would be willing to share their experience with their condition and/or dealing with the medical system. I can only describe some of the responses as heartbreaking.

For example, Lesley told me a bit about her experience with Hashimoto's thyroiditis and Graves' disease. Despite having been diagnosed with Graves for 32 years and Hashimoto's for a year and with a medical support team, life is still difficult.

"Every day is a struggle… I can't remember the last time I woke in the morning feeling refreshed and by 11 am I feel

like I've been awake for three days! Then there's the headaches and nausea... On my days off I'm so fatigued I just lay in bed all day... I try to be social but this horrendous disease dictates my life..."

Kate wrote to me about her issues with antiphospholipid antibodies, an autoimmune condition that affects blood cells. She wrote that she feels *"like a ticking time bomb... I can't think I'm so tired, sigh... I've written everything down for years and will continue doing that. I've been shocking with names for years, even places. That's become worse with the 'brain fog' and I do stumble a bit at times during conversations. It's embarrassing but I get there eventually."*

Somebody must be benefitting from this system for it to continue, but from my vantage point, it isn't the majority of people with an autoimmune condition. I think it's well and truly time that we started asking some serious questions about who our medical industries serve.

Even regulatory bodies that oversee the health industry don't come out of this unscathed. What do I mean by this? Let's look at Australia as an example. We have a relatively tightly controlled medical system. Yet even here, our regulatory bodies are largely funded by industry profits. The Therapeutic Goods Administration, which oversees all of the medications and any products that make therapeutic health claims in Australia, has a total revenue of AU$184 million. AU$169 million of that comes directly from industry (28). That's over *90%*.

Meanwhile, the National Institutes of Health is the largest public funder of biomedical research in the United States. Its primary role is to support and conduct medical research to improve health outcomes. Yet 95% of its advisory committees have been shown to have ties with food and/or pharmaceutical companies (29). This means that the vast majority of the people steering medical research and policy in the US have a vested interest in the companies' selling medications and processed foods.

Are you willing to take your medical and dietary advice from people who make a financial profit when you're sick or eat certain products?

Medicine is Sexist

I'm not going to mince my words here: the gender disparity is well documented in medicine. The vast majority of studies focus on men's medical conditions and the effects of medications on men. Yet, as Dr. Stacy Sims puts it, "Women are not small men!" (30).

Our needs differ from men's. Approximately 75% of people with autoimmune diseases are biologically female, yet the treatments and techniques used are more commonly tested in males. We don't know if they're appropriate for women (31; 32; 33).

Evidence also shows women are often seen as hypochondriacs (34; 35). Yet, according to the American Autoimmune Related Diseases Association, 40% of women with autoimmune conditions are initially dismissed. They're told they're complainers or too concerned with their health

(36). And here in Australia, at least two out of three women experience sex-based discrimination in healthcare (37).

Yvonne S., diagnosed with Hashimoto's thyroiditis earlier this year, shared her journey with me.

"For many years, I had been feeling chronically tired and dealing with persistent body, joint, and muscle aches. Despite these symptoms, my blood tests typically came back within range—except for my ferritin levels, which were always low. Even in the February results, low ferritin was noted, but no GP ever questioned this or sought to investigate its root cause. I was simply told that I had low ferritin (no shit!) and was perimenopausal (also not news). One GP even suggested I take SSRIs, promising I'd feel better in a few weeks. I declined the SSRIs and never returned to that GP."

It's not just in the primary care setting that discrimination can occur, either.

I recently completed my Masters of Counselling. Counselling is a mental health profession that prides itself on "person-centred care" (38). This means prioritising patients' concerns above all else (within legal guidelines). Yet in my course, we were taught that "psychogenic pain", pain with no obvious medical cause, happens purely in the brain as the result of emotional suffering and should be treated as such (39).

This ignores the well-established link between emotions and immune function (40). (More on this later!)

Other evidence suggests immune dysregulation may be at the heart of otherwise inexplicable chronic pain (17).

And guess who most commonly suffers from so-called psychogenic chronic pain? Women.

I can't help but wonder if my diagnostic trajectory might have been different if I had been born with a different set of reproductive organs.

We Need a Culture Shift in Medicine

Do we need a culture shift in medicine? Based on my own ongoing experience and that of my clients, I say the resounding answer is yes.

Some doctors agree. Dr. Casey Means says it's very competitive. It's more about awards and prestige than about care and empathy (41). Dr. Lissa Rankin highlights this same problem (42).

As Melanie, who has Hashimoto's thyroiditis, told me:

"Getting help in Canberra is ridiculous, Drs here will only test TSH and T4. T3 is paid for (by Medicare, Australia's publicly funded health system), *still not all will test it and generally there's no one that will prescribe it anyway.*

This highlights a major issue. Thyroid-stimulating hormone (TSH) and thyroxine (T4) are the two most commonly tested biomarkers for Hashimoto's thyroiditis. Research suggests that not everyone with Hashimoto's has TSH or T4 outside the normal range – up to 20% of people, though I suspect this number may be more (43; 44). It's only when triiodothyronine (T3) and antibodies are tested that their issues will show up. This is the reason why it took me so long to get a diagnosis of Hashimoto's because my T3 and antibodies weren't tested until I ordered those tests myself. If the medical system were set up to better support us, and if doctors listened to their patients more, I believe that many of us would get the help we sorely need much sooner.

Dr Nick Coatsworth advocates for a shift from rewarding doctors for treating patients' symptoms quickly with medications to rewarding them for helping patients understand the *cause* of their condition. This, he says, will make for a better long-term prognosis and provide more real value (16). It will enable patients to make the crucial lifestyle changes needed to realise better health outcomes.

This gets to the heart of the issue. We need to shift from a medical model that writes autoimmune diseases off as inexplicable conditions with no known root cause to one that empowers patients with the latest research findings and therapeutic advances.

People need help understanding how underlying genetic predispositions can interact with lifestyle factors and physiology to produce autoimmune diseases and what they can do on a day-to-day basis to prevent or reverse them.

If our current system can't prevent a 12.5% yearly rise in autoimmune diseases, we must question its efficacy. It's time to change the accepted standards of care. The medical model we're using to treat autoimmune diseases isn't working. It treats symptoms without restoring true health to individuals or preventing others from getting sick.

We Need to Be Empowered

I live in Victoria, Australia. Probably because of where I am, Better Health Channel often ranks towards the top of results when I do a Google search with health-related terms. This is a Victorian government website meant to provide health information to the public.

The following is an excerpt from the section on thyroid medication on its Hashimoto's thyroiditis information page.

> *"You will need to take the medication for life. Medication does not cure the condition but helps maintain normal thyroid hormone levels. The symptoms will return if thyroid medication is stopped.* (45)*"*

I hardly need to spell out how hopeless complete remission seems when you read this. But I want to reassure you that your body can heal and knows exactly how to do it under the right conditions.

When I got my diagnosis of Hashimoto's, I elected not to take medication. I had already improved my symptoms by noticing what my triggers were and learning what I could do to support my body to heal. Once I had a diagnosis, I managed complete remission within two and a half years of diagnosis.

In the 22 months since then, I've run a marathon, started and completed a master's degree and several other certifications, launched a new business, written this book, and built new and maintained existing strong social relationships. Plus, all the usual household chores, work (including running my own business), and ongoing renovations on our house.

All of these things require energy and focus. As anyone with any autoimmune disease (and especially Hashimoto's) will tell you, simply having the energy to roll out of bed each morning is a struggle when your body is under attack from its immune system.

Yet here I am, symptom-free, going full-speed ahead. Either the Victorian Government is wrong, or every single blood test or ultrasound I had that confirmed either my diagnosis or remission was wrong. I know which I think is more likely.

If I could reverse a so-called "incurable" condition without a drop of medication and go on to do all that I've done since, so can others. There's evidence in the academic literature that it's possible (46). There's plenty of anecdotal evidence as well (47).

Right now, there's a lot of change on the horizon in the American health sector. Whatever happens, it will likely affect Australian policy because we so often follow in America's footsteps. No one knows exactly what will happen yet or how the proposed changes will be realised.

But, as someone who specialises in chronic disease management and remission, I have to tell you that these changes can't come fast enough for the people I work with. Whatever you might think of him, Robert Kennedy's stance on the pharmaceutical industry's involvement in public decision-making and more holistic approaches to health and nutrition offers a tiny glimmer of hope to the people I serve.

We need reform in our medical system to not only get better diagnosis and treatment for autoimmune diseases but also to give people a future to look forward to.

Let that be our starting point, but not where the changes end.

What I Propose We Focus On

The main reason I wrote this book is to answer what I consider to be the single most important question any of us should be asking about autoimmune diseases: *why do we get them?*

We need to understand the root cause of autoimmune diseases.

If our current system can't prevent a 12.5% yearly rise in autoimmune diseases, we must question its efficacy. It's time to change the accepted standards of care. The medical model we're using to treat autoimmune disease isn't working. It treats symptoms without restoring true health to individuals or preventing others from getting sick.

It does not address the root causes of these diseases.

What I'm going to discuss is how to retrain your immune system. We can do this through natural methods that reduce the disease and its causes. I see this as a much safer way of working with autoimmune diseases. Not only is it more effective and efficient, but side effects are minimal (if there are any), and there is potential to provide long-term benefits.

My Approach is Holistic *and* Research-Backed

The approach that I take in this book is based on a similar approach that I took to reverse my autoimmune disease. The principles are the same; it has just become more refined and informed since then.

It's a systems-based approach, where I see all of the different parts of your body, their interactions, and your interactions with the external world as linked. This is what's called a systems-based or holistic approach. It's quite different from a normal Western medical approach, which is what we call "reductionist".

In my experience, reductionist approaches tend to treat symptoms of disease. Instead of treating disease *symptoms*, I'm going to show you how to use a holistic approach to treat the disease's *cause*.

If this sounds a bit out there, don't worry. You'll see peer-reviewed research referenced throughout this entire book. With a few exceptions where I will share personal experiences or anecdotes, everything I say has data behind it.

This book isn't only for those who want to take a completely natural approach. If you're on medication, you can still use what I share in this book. If anything, everything I teach you here is likely to make your medication more effective. Or enable you to slowly wean yourself off it (under careful supervision, of course!).

How the Book is Structured

To get the most out of this book, read it in full. It will give you a complete understanding of the concepts and research I explore. I realise some of what I talk about here is very dense and technical. I've tried to distil everything into the plainest language I can so that it's readily accessible to anyone.

I've split the book into three main sections.

The first section covers the biological systems behind autoimmune disease. It introduces some key concepts you need to know for the rest of the book. From this point forward, you will also find an exercise at the end of each chapter (including this one). These are optional but highly recommended. The more of these exercises you do, the more you'll learn about yourself and your autoimmune condition.

The second section discusses lifestyle factors that can cause autoimmune diseases. The exercises at the end of each chapter in this section are aimed at helping you identify problem areas in your lifestyle. You can then correct these using the tips and insights shared in the chapter. You must do this because the principles I share will form the foundations for long-term health.

The last section goes through some of the common issues that people face in the context of gene-environment interactions. It will help you identify them and address them in a way that is specifically tailored to *your* unique biology. You can do this with genetic data (there are instructions on how to get this in the book), or you can do it without. The more data you have, the easier it generally is to identify and address these kinds of issues. But if you don't want or can't afford to get it for some reason, you will still find the information presented useful.

Ready to dive in? In the next chapter, we're going to start by exploring the underlying biology and physiology involved in autoimmune diseases. It all starts with your DNA.

Exercise

Manifest your perfect day

This is the first step in the process. I don't want you to think I've gone woo-woo, but you're going to do a manifesting exercise to start with. This is to get your mind ready for change and help you set some goals for the future. It's simple but effective. I did this in 2020, not long after I found out I had Hashimoto's. I wrote down what an ideal day in my life would be like in three years. This is very similar to the miracle question I was taught to do in solutions-focused therapy but goes more in-depth.

Every morning for a couple of weeks, I would walk down to the café near where I was living and spend an hour or so on it. I went over it multiple times, trying to perfect every tiny detail. I let my imagination run wild. I didn't let myself be governed by rules about what I'd been told was and wasn't possible. Almost everything that I wrote about has since come true. I went into full remission two and a half years later. This book is one of the last things I conjured up in my mind and committed to paper to be realised. That means it's time for me to do it again and set a whole new set of goals for myself.

I've heard several podcasts and talks by self-help gurus and authors about this exercise. So, it's hard to say who to credit it to. It's likely been in use for a long time. For hundreds, if not thousands, of years. But it was probably first popularised in the West by Shakti Gawain's 1978 book, Creative Visualisation. She calls it "Day in Your Future Life" and outlines how to do it as a visualisation.

Here are the steps for visualising your perfect day, according to Gawain. While the exercise is broadly presented, the key instructions she gives for it typically include the following steps (plus a few embellishments from me):

1. Begin by finding a quiet place where you won't be disturbed. Sit or lie down comfortably, close your eyes, and take a few deep breaths to relax your body and mind.

2. Set an intention to visualise a day in your ideal future life. This day should mark the achievement of your most important goals. Set it at 1-3 years in the future. This gives time for readjustment while keeping it close enough to the present to feel tangible.

3. Imagine yourself waking up on this ideal day. Visualise every detail as vividly as you can. Include your location, your surroundings, and who you are with. Describe what you do and how you feel. Imagine going through your daily routine. You do things that show your fulfilled life. Be specific about what you see, hear, and feel. Be specific about your health, energy levels, and self-care. Go right through how you would spend an ideal day, up until the moment you go back to bed and fall asleep.

4. As you visualise, pay close attention to your emotions. Feel the happiness, contentment, and peace that come with living this ideal day. The exercise's emotional experience is crucial. It aligns your energy with the reality you want to manifest.

5. End the visualisation by expressing gratitude for the life you have envisioned. Feel thankful, as if it has already manifested. This gratitude strengthens your intent. It boosts the positive energy tied to your future life.

Gawain suggests doing this exercise often. It will reinforce the vision and keep your focus on manifesting your desired future (48). I also recommend that you write it down, like I did. Why? Because then you can go back and keep adding more details. The more details you add, the more real it feels. And the more real it feels, the more likely it is that it will come true.

The reason why this works is that it helps you clarify what you truly want for yourself (49; 50). It helps refine your values and your priorities.

But more than that, it makes what you want tangible. One of the biggest problems we have as adults is changing our habits and behaviours. We can know that something is logically a good idea based on evidence. But, if we doubt ourselves, we will question if things work for us. If you can do this exercise and make it feel real, you're giving yourself a far better chance of success. The future vision is something for you to hold onto when things get tough.

If you feel as though what you care about and want is possible, your behaviour will inevitably follow. And who knows, maybe it's also helping you send a message to the universe.

Part 1 – Understanding the Biology and Physiology Underpinning Autoimmune Diseases

Your Autoimmune Condition is Genetic but Not Inevitable

"...the vast majority of people come into this world with genes that should enable them to live a happy and healthy life."

Bruce Lipton, *The Biology of Belief*

I suspected a fundamental flaw in myself when I bombed out of university at 19 due to anxiety, followed by depression. It seemed I was somehow different from my parents and siblings.

They were all stable and competent. I, on the other hand, couldn't remember being free from anxiety for any significant period since I was a kid without taking some pretty drastic measures to numb myself and quiet my mind. I wondered if I had been unlucky in the genetic lottery, my parents' genes combining in some completely novel way.

This thought terrified me. What if I could never be happy? What if my genes doomed me to depression and mental health issues my entire life?

But, as I discovered later, genes are only part of the picture.

Understanding Genetic Inheritance Patterns

Throughout this chapter, I'm going to give an overview of genetics and their role in autoimmune disease. This is important for understanding their root cause since they are heritable conditions. This means that if your parents or close relatives have an autoimmune disease, there's a greater chance of you developing an autoimmune disease.

However, as I'll soon explain, this doesn't mean you're pre-destined to get an autoimmune disease. There's nuance to the genetic inheritance of autoimmune conditions. What I'm going to reveal in this chapter is crucial to understanding the mechanisms underpinning the genetic complexities of autoimmune conditions and what you can do to manage or reverse them.

If you feel that you already have a solid understanding of current genetics research, you can skip this section, though I wouldn't recommend skipping the entire chapter. Just jump through to the methylation and detoxification section.

For those less familiar with genetics, let's go through a brief overview of how genetic inheritance works.

I'm sure you know who we are depends on our genes. Genes are segments of Deoxyribonucleic Acid (DNA). They contain the instructions for building proteins (51).

Proteins are essential molecules that perform many functions in the body. They're like the body's workhorses. If you lack them, have the wrong types, or they aren't working well, your body won't be as responsive to the demands you place on it. You won't be feeling at your most vibrant or optimal.

Proteins underpin everything we do.

There's a complex two-way relationship between gene function and protein formation. Your DNA relies on having enough and the right types of proteins to express itself and, therefore, to produce more proteins (52). Gene expression is the process by which information from a gene is used to build functional molecules like proteins, which perform numerous vital roles within cells. Gene expression occurs in two steps.

The first begins in the cell's nucleus, where specific proteins initiate the copying of a gene's DNA sequence into a molecule called messenger RNA (mRNA). This step, known as transcription, relies on various proteins to ensure that the right genes are expressed at the right time.

Once mRNA is produced, it exits the nucleus and travels to the cell's cytoplasm to complete the second step. Here, ribosomes—structures also composed of proteins and RNA—read the mRNA sequence and translate it into a chain of amino acids, ultimately folding it into a functional protein. These newly formed proteins then perform essential functions: they can act as enzymes to speed up biochemical reactions, structural components of the cell, or regulators of gene expression itself.

Therefore, gene expression not only requires proteins to initiate and regulate transcription and translation but also produces proteins that influence cellular structure, metabolism, and gene activity, forming a cycle that is essential to cell function and organism health.

For instance, some proteins, like collagen and keratin, provide structural support, while others act as enzymes, aiding metabolism and digestion. Signalling proteins, like hormones and antibodies, help cells communicate and defend against infections. Regulatory proteins control gene expression and cell functions (53). The instructions for making all these proteins are encoded by our genes.

You get one copy of most of your genes from each parent (54). Your genetic blueprint is made up of pairs of chromosomes. These are long, paired strands of DNA that contain different genes. There are 23 chromosomes in the human genome. Each parent contributes one chromosome in each chromosome pair to their offspring. So, you get one chromosome in the pair from each parent, which is how you inherit roughly 50% of your genes from each of them.

You have between 20 000–25 000 genes spread across your 23 chromosomes. Each of these is located at a different locus. Locus is the term used in genetics for specifying the location of a gene. Loci (plural for locus) are specific positions on chromosomes where genes or genetic markers are located, and they play a key role in genetic inheritance by determining where particular traits or variations are encoded.

But not all genes have only variant; many have multiple variants, which work in very similar ways but with some slight differences. In total, you have between 30 000–40 000 loci for functional genes.

On top of that, because chromosomes are made of twin strands, you have two different alleles at each locus. Allele is the name given to the specific copy of a single gene or a gene variant that you inherited from either your (biological) mother or father.

Your genotype consists of your specific genes, regardless of whether they express themselves or not. Gene expression creates your phenotype. It's the visible or expressed trait for a characteristic, which can range from your looks to your metabolism.

In what's known as the Mendelian pattern of genetic inheritance, one allele of a gene is more dominant than any of the others. This version of the gene will express itself if it's present. We call this the dominant allele, while other alleles of the same gene are recessive in comparison. If you have both a dominant allele and a recessive allele, the dominant gene will be the one that gets expressed. If you have two recessive copies of a gene, you'll express the trait linked to the recessive one.

In BIO101, I remember learning the classic example of the phenotype for eye colour. Eyes come in three main colours—brown, green, and blue. Brown (B) eyes prevail, a dominant characteristic, whereas blue (b) eyes are less common because they're recessive. This is an example of monogenic inheritance. It means one set of genes determines the phenotype.

If a person inherits a dominant brown eye allele from either parent, they will have brown eyes. The dominant gene overpowers the recessive one. For example, both BB and Bb genotypes result in brown eyes.

To have blue eyes, an individual must inherit two recessive alleles (bb), one from each parent. An absence of a dominant allele allows for the expression of the recessive trait.

Green eyes are an exception to the rule. They arise from the combined effect of more than one gene, inherited in what's known as a polygenic pattern. One of the key genes involved is the OCA2 gene, which influences the amount of melanin produced in the iris.

Green eyes occur when there is a moderate amount of melanin, more than in blue eyes but less than in brown eyes. Different alleles (variants) of these genes can produce green eyes.

So, to have green eyes, a person inherits alleles that create an intermediate level of melanin. Green eyes are less common than brown but more common than blue in some populations. This is due to genetic complexity.

I've put all of the terms that I just outlined into a table below. Hopefully this helps simplify and clarify all of these terms for you.

Genetic Terms

Term	Meaning
Chromosome	Long DNA molecule that contains part or all the genetic material of an organism.
Locus	The specific, fixed position on a chromosome where a particular gene or genetic marker is located.
Genotype	What genes you have.
Phenotype	What genes you express.
Mendelian genetics	A pattern of gene expression based on dominant and recessive genes.
Dominant allele	A gene variant that expresses its trait even when a different allele is present at the same locus.
Recessive allele	A gene variant that only expresses its trait when no dominant allele is present at the same locus.
Monogenic inheritance	When one gene is enough to determine a trait on its own.
Polygenic inheritance	The process by which multiple genes contribute to a single trait, resulting in a broad range of phenotypic outcomes.

I won't go into more detail on genetic inheritance because it's a whole discipline, and we could get bogged down in it. You don't need to know everything there is to know about genetics, but the basics covered above are going to come in handy as you learn more about the genetic aspects of autoimmune diseases in this book.

Epigenetics and Malleable Gene Expression

When I was studying my science degree at university, I was taught that genes were deterministic. The genes you got were the ones you were stuck with and there was no changing it.

This is only part of the truth. We now know that many genes are far more malleable in their expression than was originally thought. This means you don't express all your inherited genes from your parents. Instead, external bioelectric signals can activate specific pathways in the cell. This triggers chemical processes that turn certain genes on or off.

A fascinating example of how we learnt more about this was a study conducted by researchers Tseng and Levin in 2012. They were investigating how bioelectric signals impact gene expression, development, and regeneration in tadpoles.

They manipulated electrical gradients across cell membranes and found that even though the DNA stayed the same, gene expression was altered. This included genes related to eye formation and tail regeneration, causing tails to develop eye-like features. Because the experiment was conducted in a controlled environment and other factors were controlled for, the researchers concluded that not only can bioelectric signals override genetic instructions, they are essential for normal development. This opens the door to potential regenerative medicine therapies that target bioelectric pathways (55).

Before you get your hopes up: regenerative medicine can't yet heal autoimmune diseases caused by antibody damage. Yet, some strategies and supplements can trigger healing pathways in a similar way. More on this later in the book.

Bioelectric signals allow your body's cells to communicate, regulating important processes like gene expression, muscle movement, heartbeat, and digestion. These signals are controlled by neurons and involve ion channels, cell membranes, and the regulation of hormones and neurotransmitters. They also affect brain activity, influencing mood, thoughts, and behaviour by altering hormone levels (56).

For example, the nervous system coordinates the signals that tell your arm where to move to catch a ball by sending bioelectric signals. Its primary role is to coordinate responses to events, both internal and external (57).

Your nervous system is constantly working. This means your genes get constant signals about what to do. Sometimes, it's telling them to keep on doing what they're doing. Other times, it's telling them to stop because whatever protein they produce is no longer needed. And sometimes, it'll signal that they need to start doing something new pronto and make a different protein to meet a new challenge.

What this means is that your genes are constantly receiving signals, and adjusting to help meet the demands of whatever situation you're in.

Scientists study these changes in a field called "epigenetics" (58). It examines how cells alter gene expression to produce traits. As demonstrated in the tadpole tail experiment, these changes happen without changing the underlying DNA sequence, only which genes are turned on or off.

Mechanisms Governing Epigenetics

Three primary mechanisms govern epigenetic modifications:

1. **DNA methylation** is like a tiny tag that tells certain parts of your genetic code whether to be active or quiet. It works by adding a small chemical called a methyl group to specific spots in your DNA. When these spots get tagged, it usually means nearby genes won't do their jobs. When the tag is removed, they're free to express themselves again. This

tagging process is vital for controlling your genes. It is most important during growth, when cells change type, and in diseases like autoimmune disease (59).

2. **Histone modifications** are tiny switches on the proteins that package your DNA. You can activate or deactivate these switches by adding different chemical tags to the proteins. A switch's activation allows nearby genes to be readily accessed and utilized. These changes are important. They help cells respond quickly to environmental shifts by turning genes on or off as needed (60).

3. **Non-coding RNAs** are molecular messengers that don't make proteins. Instead, they control how the cell *uses* your genes. Some, like microRNAs, can stick to messenger RNAs, stopping them from making proteins. Some long non-coding RNAs can talk to the proteins that package your DNA. They help turn genes on or off (61).

These epigenetic mechanisms work together to regulate gene expression. They respond to developmental signals, environmental stimuli, and physiological processes (62). Each mechanism has its own roles, specific to certain circumstances.

The next thing to understand is how developmental signals impact gene expression. For example, your eye colour likely stayed the same after nine months because it's a more fixed trait, influenced by developmental signals (63). These signals guide gene expression, especially during critical development periods. Critical periods vary by trait, with most taking place before birth, when organs and systems are forming and are most sensitive to external influences (64).

These early stages lay the foundation for our basic human structures.

Most of you won't have been born with an autoimmune disease. It's something that has developed later in life. This is because genes involved in autoimmune disease are governed by environmental cues and physiological processes, rather than developmental signals (65; 66).

In fact, around 85-90% of your genes are governed by epigenetic processes. Only 10-15% are associated with developmental signals and critical periods (67). In the immune system, there is slightly less malleability, with 25-30% of genes involved in immune function highly conserved, meaning they are fairly stable in their activity (68). This is important for a couple of reasons. For a start, they play an important role in metabolism and energy production. You need these genes to be working at all times to function at a basic level. Secondly, it provides you with a baseline defence system against threats like pathogens. However, these genes aren't the ones directly involved in the production of antibodies in autoimmune disease, nor do they cause aches, pains, and fatigue under normal circumstances.

This is pertinent for two reasons for those with autoimmune disease (69). Firstly, it means that we can turn off the genetic part of autoimmune disease. Unlike developmental genes such as eye colour, the genes involved express themselves flexibly. This lets you, the organism, adapt to your changing world and increases your chances of surviving environmental challenges.

Secondly, autoimmune diseases usually develop later in life. This suggests multiple gene involvement, as most critical periods have passed. Children can develop an autoimmune disease, but it's rare. Age is the best predictor of autoimmune disease risk (70). A whole-system dysfunction takes time because it depends on the activation of several genes, not just one (71).

Researchers have found this with autoimmune diseases. Like eye colour, they are mostly polygenic conditions, meaning they are influenced by more than one gene, with a few are exceptions (72). Many genes lead to their development and progression; there's not one single genetic switch that leads to chronic inflammation and the production of antibodies that attack the self. The symptoms you experience are orchestrated by the combined effects of multiple genes.

This makes it trickier to reverse them because you need to stop more than one gene from expressing itself.

But it can provide a buffer against getting those symptoms again. It's not like flicking one switch and then, bam! You're sick again. It's generally a process of decline. If you know the signs, you can fix it. You can reverse it before it's too late.

It also means that autoimmune disease can occur on a sliding scale of severity depending on how many genes involved in the immune response are expressing themselves (73). At its worst, with many autoimmune genes active, you feel terrible and can't function. At its mildest, you might notice a slight niggle or impairment in your energy levels.

Genetics in the Context of Autoimmune Disease

There are many genes linked to autoimmune disease. Some of them are specific to a single type of autoimmune disease, while some are linked to a much wider range of autoimmune diseases.

Perhaps the most widely studied of these broadly implicated genes are the HLA genes (74). They regulate how the body recognises and responds to foreign substances and play a crucial role in determining how the body identifies pathogens versus identification of the self.

This is due to what's known as mutations in the gene. A mutation is a change in the DNA sequence of a gene, which can alter the function or regulation of that gene and may lead to variations in an organism's traits or health. This alteration can occur due to errors in DNA replication, exposure to environmental factors, or inherited changes from biological parents (75).

Certain mutations in these genes make it more likely that the immune system will recognise the self as foreign and make an attack on your organs and tissues. Mutations aren't necessarily bad—sometimes, they can be a good thing. As you'll soon learn, there have historically been advantages to having these versions of these genes. In modern times, though, their presence can be devastating.

But just having these genes is no guarantee of having an autoimmune disease.

For example, 90-95% of people with celiac disease have the *HLA-DQ2* allele, and most of the rest carry *HLA-DQ8*. Yet only 1-3% of people with these genes actually develop celiac disease (76).

Likewise, variants of the *HLA-DRB1* gene are strongly associated with rheumatoid arthritis. About 60–70% of RA patients have one of these HLA variants, but they are also present in 20–30% of healthy individuals (77).

Even in Type 1 Diabetes, which is regarded as the most heritable polygenic autoimmune condition, only a small proportion of carriers of HLA alleles associated with the condition develop it (78).

This makes it hard to predict your risk of autoimmune diseases from a genetic test. Also, using genetic tests for diagnosis is difficult. Not all gene tests will check the thousands of genes linked to autoimmune diseases. Plus, if there's no family history of autoimmune disease, it can be difficult to know what to test for.

Furthermore, most genetic testing has limitations. It only looks at *parts* of the human genome. While whole-genome testing is now available, it's expensive. We likely have to wait a few years for affordable tests. Then, it will take even longer, years if not decades, to understand all the genes in autoimmune diseases (79; 80).

Methylation and Detoxification Genes Hold More Answers

A better way to predict your chances of getting an autoimmune disease is a gene test that evaluates genes involved in methylation and detoxification. Detoxification is an umbrella term for processes undertaken constantly by organs like your liver, kidneys, gallbladder, and intestines to remove waste and harmful compounds from your body. We're going to discuss why genes involved in detoxification may be important in just a moment, but first, I want to explain methylation and why it's significant.

As explained before, genes are epigenetically modified in three ways. This is done via methylation, histone modifications, and non-coding RNA regulation. These mechanisms lead to genes either being expressed or silenced.

As you can probably infer, methylation genes play a role in regulating epigenetic expression. We know a lot more about methylation pathways and genes associated with them than we do the other two mechanisms of epigenetic regulation. There are a couple of reasons for this. One is that it has been a historical research focus due to its role in developmental biology and cancer (59). Another is that technology to research and assess methylation pathways has advanced more quickly (81).

This isn't to say that histone modifications and non-coding RNA regulation aren't important. But we know far less about them and their role in autoimmune diseases. This makes methylation a crucial pathway to focus on in understanding the epigenetic underpinnings of autoimmune disease – at least for now.

Some genes make enzymes for this pathway to work well. However, some people have mutations in genes involved in methylation, which impair their function. As a result, people who have these mutations that lead to genes not working as well have an increased risk of autoimmune disease (82).

This is because they inappropriately suppress or permit certain immune genes to activate. In autoimmune diseases, hypomethylation is common. It means that *not enough* methylation has occurred, so it isn't silencing genes involved in the immune response in the way it should (83; 84). For instance, in rheumatoid arthritis, cells called synovial fibroblasts in the joint capsule's inner layer have shown hypomethylation (85).

Researchers have also found that hypermethylation can be a problem in autoimmune diseases (86). As the name suggests, hypermethylation is when *too much* methylation has taken place. Too many genes have been silenced when they ought not to have been.

In either case, dysregulated methylation plays a role in autoimmune disease. It's a strong contender for an epigenetic cause.

Sometimes, a gene has more than one variant involved in a specific process. These different variants of a gene are called polymorphisms.

For example, the MTHFR gene helps with methylation. It has over 50 different known polymorphisms but the two most well-researched problematic polymorphisms are C677T and A1298C. Both are linked to autoimmune conditions, including Hashimoto's Thyroiditis (87). These polymorphisms have similar but distinct effects. If someone has two copies of C677T, they produce only about 30% of the MTHFR enzyme. Two copies of A1298C reduce production by 20-40% (88). Having one copy of either polymorphism can reduce enzyme production. Having both can worsen the effect, as their activity compounds.

What this means is that methylation genes work differently to Mendelian genetics. One allele isn't dominant over another. They depend on the combined impact of multiple genes (89; 90). They're *polygenic*, just like green eye colour and most autoimmune diseases. The outcome is the level of enzyme production, which is determined by input from many genes.

On top of that, there are several different genes involved in the methylation pathway. We're going to look at it in more detail later on, but having mutations that reduce enzyme production or stability in any of the genes involved in methylation can increase your risk of developing an autoimmune condition. This makes them worth understanding and studying.

The other genes well worth paying attention to are those involved in detoxification. Polymorphisms or mutations in genes involved in detoxification processes are also linked to autoimmune diseases (91; 92). These genes produce proteins that prevent harmful substances from building up in the body

(93; 94). We'll dive into "harmful substances" and detoxification in the next section so don't worry if you're not sure what I mean by this right now.

Detoxification pathways and genes that play a role in them are also tightly linked to methylation, which I'll explain soon as well.

The table below denotes some examples of genes involved in methylation and detoxification pathways shown to be implicated in autoimmune diseases.

Gene	Type	Effect
MTHFR	Methylation	Common variants, such as C677T and A1298C, reduce enzyme efficiency and are associated with elevated homocysteine levels, which may contribute to inflammation and immune dysregulation. Research has linked these variants to an increased risk for autoimmune diseases like Behcet's disease, ankylosing spondylitis, and multiple sclerosis (82).
MTR & MTRR	Methylation	Mutations in these genes, such as MTR A2756G and MTRR A66G, are associated with impaired methylation and have been linked to autoimmune conditions like

		multiple sclerosis and rheumatoid arthritis (95).
COMT	Intermediate between methylation & detoxification	COMT is involved in the breakdown of catecholamines, which include dopamine, epinephrine, and norepinephrine. The Val158Met mutation in COMT affects enzyme function and may impact stress responses and inflammation regulation. Elevated catecholamine levels, resulting from COMT dysfunction, are linked to heightened immune response and have been associated with autoimmune diseases (96).
CBS	Intermediate between methylation & detoxification	CBS is essential in the transsulphuration pathway for homocysteine metabolism. Mutations, such as 844ins68 in CBS, can lead to high homocysteine levels, linked with increased inflammation and higher autoimmune disease risk (97).
GST	Detoxification	GST genes, including GSTP1, GSTM1, and GSTT1, are involved in detoxification pathways. These

		genes help detoxify free radicals and environmental toxins. Variants like GSTP1 Ile/Val, Val/Val and GSTM1 null mutation can reduce glutathione efficiency, increasing oxidative stress, increasing risk for lupus and Sjögren's syndrome (98).
SOD2	Detoxification	SOD2 mutations affect mitochondrial antioxidant defences. Variants like Ala16Val in SOD2 can impair superoxide dismutation, leading to mitochondrial dysfunction and oxidative stress and has been linked to lupus (99).
NQO1	Detoxification	NQO1 is part of the body's detoxification system, crucial for protecting cells against oxidative stress. The NQO1 C609T polymorphism reduces enzyme activity, making individuals more susceptible to environmental toxins and oxidative stress, contributing to autoimmune disease development (100).

One other thing to note is that these genes can affect how medications work. They can also influence medication side effects (101; 102). So, it's well worth getting to know what yours are, even if you're planning on taking a medicated route to manage your condition rather than doing things naturally. This can enable you to work with your doctor or specialist to choose the medication that's most likely to work with the least side effects.

You're not doomed if you have genetic issues with methylation or detoxification, though (103).

The changes they cause aren't necessarily a problem unless other factors arise. There can be problems when your need for the enzymes they code for increases. The circumstances that can increase their need is where we're going in the next chapter.

Task

Getting Your Genes Tested

If you're curious about your genetics and can afford it, getting some insight into your unique genetics can be one of the most empowering things you can do. If I could go back in time and go through my journey with Hashimoto's all over again, this is exactly where I would start. It's a brilliant way to find the causes of your conditions. Getting your methylation and detoxification panels is very powerful. It can help you support proper epigenetic expression. It can also help downregulate genes in your immune and antioxidant defence systems. And they will never change like blood work does. You'll have those results for life. They will be valuable if any health issues arise.

Many online services offer genetic testing. Or you can find a practitioner like me to help you. I often use Ancestry with clients for genetic testing. It's cheap and analyses a wide range of genes. Most importantly, it includes most methylation and detoxification genes. 23andMe is also reportedly excellent and tests a wide range of genes.

These sites don't analyse health, though. You need to download the raw data from the websites and then run it through an analyser. Many free or cheap analysis tools exist online. My favourite free tool is Genetic Genie. It does a fairly thorough methylation and detox analysis.

I now have an online tool for gene analysis as well. It provides you with a comprehensive report, flagging genes that present major issues, especially if other genes that interact with them are present. It also provides broad nutrition guidelines as well as a more personalised nutritional approach based on your genes, including any supplements that may be helpful and quantities. It also explains how certain genes work synergistically to create states of poor health. You can find out more about it on my website. It's called "Eat for Your Genes".

If you do get your genes tested, you may also find the information valuable later in the final section of this book. But don't worry if you can't afford to do it or don't want to – I've made sure that everyone can access the information they need to better manage or reverse their immune condition in this book.

Chapter Summary

- Genes provide the instructions for building proteins, which underpin everything that happens in the body.
- You (mostly) get one copy of each gene from your biological mother and biological father, meaning that we have two copies of each gene.
- There can be multiple variations of each gene: the dominant gene is the one that's usually expressed, although it can sometimes be a little more complicated.
- Epigenetics is the field of science that studies these changes in gene expression that occur without alterations to the underlying gene sequence.
- The three mechanisms by which epigenetic changes to genes occur are called methylation, histone modifications, and non-coding RNA.
- Some genes, like those involved in critical periods of development, are less malleable than others, which respond to changes in physiology and the external environment.
- Autoimmune diseases are caused by more malleable genes, so they can be turned on and off.
- Autoimmune diseases are mostly polygenic conditions, meaning that multiple genes are involved. This makes them harder to reverse but also harder to get than if just one gene was involved.
- Autoimmune diseases exist on a sliding scale, meaning that there are differences in symptom severity. The more severe your symptoms, the more

genes that contribute to the condition are likely being expressed, and vice versa.

- Because there are many genes involved in autoimmune conditions and many different autoimmune conditions, it can be hard to predict based on broad-spectrum gene testing which autoimmune diseases a person is likely to develop or to use gene testing as a primary diagnostic tool.
- Studying genes involved in methylation and detoxification is a more viable alternative, as dysregulated methylation has been implicated in autoimmune diseases, as has dysregulated detoxification. They hold clues about what's gone wrong with your immune system and what you can do to resolve it.

An Overactive Immune System as a Response to a Distress Signal

"Once stressors accumulate beyond the threshold of tolerance, their combined impact renders the response system dysfunctional… it's imperative never to cross that threshold."

Ori Hofmekler, *The Seven Principles of Stress*

Looking back to when I got sick with Hashimoto's, I see it wasn't one thing that made me unwell. It was a myriad of things that pushed my body beyond its limit. As you'll begin to understand throughout this book, it's likely to have been the same for you.

Long-term illnesses take on distinct forms in each person. There are many types of chronic diseases. But they all come down to one thing: your redox potential. This includes autoimmune diseases but also things like cancer, metabolic syndrome, and allergies.

Redox potential describes the balance between oxidants, or reactive oxygen species (ROS), and antioxidants in the body. It is key to cellular homeostasis and health.

When this balance is disrupted, oxidants outnumber antioxidants. This causes a condition called oxidative stress.

Oxidative stress causes most chronic health conditions. This chapter explores the relationship between redox potential, oxidative stress, and autoimmune diseases.

Reactive Species and Antioxidants

Reactive species (RS) are various reactive compounds that act within the body and contain oxygen or nitrogen. They're chemically reactive molecules or ions that contain unpaired electrons or a high energy state, making them highly reactive and prone to interact with other molecules, often by accepting or donating electrons.

The most abundant and often highly reactive of them are ROS. They can easily accept electrons from other molecules, leading to oxidative reactions that can modify cellular structures, including proteins, lipids, and DNA. Superoxide radicals, hydrogen peroxide, nitrous oxide, and hydroxyl radicals are common ROS in cells. You don't need to remember them, though.

What you do need to remember is that these molecules play a role in signalling pathways. At low levels, they induce hormesis, an adaptive response to low stress. Hormesis triggers changes that help us meet future challenges (104; 105). These include creating new cells and assigning their functions. They also control apoptosis, or programmed cell death, to make way for new cells.

Additionally, they act as signals to the immune system, activating immune responses to pathogen invasion (106). The immune system also uses them as weapons against pathogens (107). They serve as signals triggering growth, renewal, and defence responses. ROS are vital to the processes that keep your cells (and you!) functioning, so they are not in and of themselves a bad thing.

But, in large quantities, they are problematic. They damage the functional components of cells. They also disrupt bioelectric signalling pathways within and between cells (108; 109).

This is where the antioxidant defence system comes in. Antioxidants are molecules that stabilise ROS, making them less reactive. This neutralises them, preventing them from being able to cause damage to the cell. In a healthy person, the body's antioxidants carefully control the concentration of ROS, keeping them within manageable levels. Antioxidants include enzymes like superoxide dismutase, catalase, and glutathione peroxidase. They also include non-enzymatic antioxidants, like vitamins C and E. They scavenge and neutralise excess RS, making them harmless (108).

Oxidative Stress and Methylation

We all generate ROS as by-products of normal cell metabolism. We can also ingest or absorb them from the external environment.

During oxidative stress, the production, ingestion, or absorption of ROS exceeds the ability of antioxidant defences to scavenge and neutralise them effectively (108). There's an imbalance in the system.

This causes ROS to build up in cells. It leads to oxidative damage to lipids, proteins, and DNA. This impairs bioelectric signalling (110; 111).

For example, cholesterol is a form of lipid vital for healthy cell membranes. It forms a permeable barrier, controlling molecular traffic in and out of the cell. Oxidative damage to cholesterol can disrupt their function by altering the fluidity of cell membranes. This impairs bioelectrical cell signalling and membrane transport. The result? Altered gene expression (112).

Oxidative stress causes the upregulation of immune system genes. This means that genes involved in the immune response are turned on in response to oxidative stress. In the context of autoimmune disease, this is a key reason for hypo- and hypermethylation (*too little* or *too much* methylation), which we discussed in the last chapter on genetics (113).

There are a couple of means by which oxidative stress can impair proper methylation. ROS can damage substances that methylate DNA, disrupting methylation processes (113). Oxidative stress also depletes a substance called S-adenosylmethionine (SAM), which is necessary for methylation to occur (114; 115). Additionally, oxidative stress can turn off genes that produce methylation substances. The body then has less capacity to respond adaptively to cues. As a result, genes involved in the immune response become active when they shouldn't be, while others that regulate immune activity can be silenced.

ROS aren't all bad news for methylation, though. They can make parts of DNA more accessible for methylation. This *increases* the expression of tumour suppressor genes (116). Thus, stress-induced changes in methylation can lower cancer risk. This highlights the dual role that ROS play in health and disease.

In small amounts, ROS can help us. They increase the expression of genes that regulate the immune response. This includes genes linked to autoimmune disease. But, at levels that cause oxidative stress, they can lead to an overactive immune system. This sparks the onset of autoimmune diseases.

Now you know a bit about gene expression changes in the context of autoimmune disease, let's discuss what causes oxidative stress.

Mitochondrial Dysfunction

Oxidative stress is especially relevant to the immune response. It can come from many sources, both internal and external. But malfunctioning mitochondria are the biggest source of oxidative stress in the body.

Mitochondria are tiny organelles in almost all your cells,e (literally) little cells within your cells. They perform many specialised functions, but they're most well-known as being the cell's powerhouses. They take food and turn it into a usable energy called adenosine triphosphate (ATP). ATP fuels everything we do.

Here's a simple explanation of how this happens. Mitochondria produce energy by breaking down nutrients like sugars and fats. These nutrients are processed through pathways like the citric acid cycle (Krebs cycle). It generates molecules that carry bioelectric energy as electrons. These electrons then pass through a series of protein complexes in the mitochondria's inner membrane. This creates a flow of charged particles called the electron transport chain. It produces ATP (117).

Metabolism generates ROS at this point. It's during the electron transport chain. Inefficiencies in the process allow electrons to "leak" and form superoxide. This can then produce other types of ROS (118).

We used to think that mitochondria only produced energy. At least, that's what my university course taught me. We now know that mitochondria also help with other processes, including everything from regulating gene expression to brain function. Their role is far more than just energy production (119; 120; 121).

You can probably guess that when these little guys aren't working too well, which we call "mitochondrial dysfunction", they cause all sorts of problems. Perhaps the most obvious one is a state of energy production that is less efficient than normal. More ROS and less ATP are produced. Not ideal.

Mitochondrial dysfunction can arise from several factors. The three main causes are energetic excess, oxidative stress, and faulty mitochondrial death and regeneration. Let's look at each of these in a little more detail.

1. **Energetic excess**, often from overnutrition or metabolic imbalances, can overwhelm mitochondria. This leads to inefficient energy production and increased ROS. Under normal circumstances, mitochondria can clear ROS quickly, sometimes instantly. They do this by producing antioxidants. This keeps things running smoothly and maintains redox balance, the balance between ROS and antioxidants. When there's

excess energy, metabolism becomes less efficient. It leaks more electrons than normal. The antioxidant defence system fails to cope, and ROS accumulate. They can damage mitochondrial DNA, proteins, and lipids. This causes oxidative stress and impairs mitochondrial function (122).

2. **Direct oxidative stress** from sources external to the body can also damage mitochondria. We'll discuss the sources of ROS that lead to oxidative stress in more detail later. For now, here's a quick overview of what happens when they encounter mitochondria. The first thing they do is disrupt the mitochondrial membranes that enclose parts of the mitochondria. The role of the mitochondrial membrane is to selectively allow molecules in and out, helping to regulate the internal environment. This is vital for proper mitochondrial function. Once the membrane loses its integrity, ROS can enter and harm parts of the mitochondria, impairing energy production. This results in less energy and more mitochondrial ROS production (123).

3. **Mitophagy** is the process of removing faulty mitochondria and recycling their parts. If this process is impaired, it can contribute to mitochondrial dysfunction. For example, if there is excess energy in the cell, the mitochondria will work faster to produce more energy but spend less time maintaining their parts via mitophagy. Eventually, the mitochondrion may become damaged beyond repair. But, if energy excess is ongoing, the cell will continue to use the damaged

mitochondrion. Then, mitophagy doesn't happen. This can lead to more mistakes and, thus, more ROS. Impaired mitophagy causes damaged mitochondria to build up in cells. This worsens oxidative stress and disrupts cellular function (124).

A buildup of ROS can also impair mitochondrial **biogenesis**, which is the process of making new, healthy mitochondria. ROS near where energy is produced can harm mitochondrial DNA, causing changes to important proteins involved in making new mitochondria. They make it harder for the DNA to copy itself and create new mitochondria. In addition, ROS can switch on certain pathways in cells that react to stress. These pathways can slow the creation of new mitochondria (124; 125).

There's one other reason why mitochondria make more ROS. They're emitted to inform cell components that they're struggling and need help. ROS aren't just produced by accident; they're also a distress signal (126).

These mechanisms highlight a feedback loop between oxidative stress and mitochondrial dysfunction. Oxidative stress from external sources can be damaging. But mitochondrial dysfunction damages the cell *from within*. It provides the conditions for further oxidative stress to develop. What's more, the more stress mitochondria are under, the more likely it is they'll produce additional ROS as signalling molecules. This is a key point that I want you to keep in mind for later on, because it will help make sense of everything else I share with you.

Mitochondria are vital to so many processes in the body that their reduced energy production and ROS generation can have serious flow-on effects. The entire body suffers when mitochondria aren't working properly. Mitochondrial dysfunction is now seen as the key cause of aging and chronic diseases underpinned by oxidative stress (127). This includes autoimmune diseases.

We've briefly discussed how oxidative stress can upregulate immune response genes. In the next chapter, we're going to explore the immune system in more detail.

Exercise

If you have an autoimmune disease, then you almost certainly are experiencing oxidative stress. This means that there's a mismatch between ROS production or ingestion and your ability to detox.

How much oxidative stress you have compared to someone else with an autoimmune disease will vary, though. Right now, as we're just starting this book, it will be helpful for you to assess your oxidative stress levels. Keep track of your results somewhere because we're going to come back to this later.

Oxidative Stress Quiz

Activity: Assessing Your Oxidative Stress Level

The following exercise is designed to help you reflect on lifestyle factors and symptoms that may indicate oxidative stress in your body. Oxidative stress occurs when there's an imbalance between reactive species and antioxidants, leading to potential cellular damage.

Instructions
Rate yourself on a scale from 1 to 5 for each statement, where:
1 = Never
2 = Rarely
3 = Sometimes
4 = Often
5 = Always

At the end, tally your score to get an idea of your potential oxidative stress level.

1. I frequently experience high levels of stress (work, family, or personal).
2. I don't get at least 7-8 hours of sleep per night.
3. I have a diet high in processed foods, sugars, and vegetable/seed oils.
4. I don't consume fruits and vegetables regularly (less than 5 servings a day).
5. I rarely eat red meat or seafood (less than 7 servings/week) and don't supplement for the essential micronutrients they contain.
6. I don't exercise or move my body regularly (less than 3 times a week).
7. I smoke or am frequently exposed to second-hand smoke.
8. I consume alcohol more than 2-3 times a week.

9. I am regularly exposed to environmental toxins (e.g., pollution, chemicals, etc.).
10. I frequently skip meals or rely on fast food/processed snacks.
11. I often feel fatigued or low on energy, even after sleeping.
12. I get frequent headaches or migraines.
13. I have digestive issues, such as bloating or irregular bowel movements.
14. My skin looks dull, dry, or shows early signs of aging (e.g., fine lines, wrinkles).
15. I often experience joint pain or stiffness.
16. I get sick often or find that it takes me longer to recover from illness.
17. I have difficulty concentrating or experience frequent brain fog.
18. I experience shortness of breath or heart palpitations.
19. I notice my mood fluctuating, often feeling anxious or irritable.
20. I have allergies or food intolerances.

Results

18-36: Low Risk of Oxidative Stress

You're likely maintaining a balance between free radicals and antioxidants. Keep supporting your health with a good diet, exercise, sleep, a healthy environment, and stress management.

37-54: Moderate Risk of Oxidative Stress

Some aspects of your lifestyle or symptoms might indicate a higher oxidative load. Keep an eye out for improvements you can make to your lifestyle throughout this book.

55+: High Risk of Oxidative Stress
You may be experiencing significant oxidative stress. This can increase your risk of chronic diseases. The information contained in the rest of this book will be highly relevant to you.

Chapter Summary

- Redox potential is a term used to describe the balance between oxidants and *anti*oxidants.
- Reactive oxygen species (ROS) are chemically reactive compounds that contain oxygen and act as oxidants in the body.
- ROS play important roles in cell growth, development, and defence when present in small quantities. In larger quantities, they can damage cell components and disrupt bioelectric signalling pathways between and within cells.
- Antioxidants are molecules that stabilise ROS, preventing them from causing damage.
- When the rate of ROS production, ingestion, or absorption exceeds the capacity of the antioxidant defence system to neutralise them, a state of oxidative stress ensues.
- Damage to cells from oxidative stress alters gene expression, including induction of hypo and hypermethylation.

- Hypo and hypermethylation can increase the expression of genes involved in the immune response.
- The most important source of oxidative stress in chronic disease states is dysfunctional mitochondria.
- Mitochondria are responsible for, among other things, cellular metabolism, the conversion of energy in food to ATP, a form of energy that the cell can readily use to fuel activities.
- A side effect of metabolism is ROS production.
- Mitochondrial dysfunction occurs when there is significantly more ROS production due to inefficiencies in the metabolic process at the expense of ATP production.
- There are three main mechanisms by which mitochondrial dysfunction arises: energetic excess in the mitochondria, direct oxidative stress to the mitochondria, and impaired mitochondrial death and regeneration processes.
- Each of these processes operates synergistically with the others, contributing to further mitochondrial dysfunction.

When an Adaptive Response Goes Wrong

"The strongest people are not those who show strength in front of the world but those who fight and win battles that others do not know anything about."

Jonathon Harnisch

Autoimmune diseases are often hidden and unobserved by the onlooker. At my sickest, many were surprised to discover I was feeling unwell. From their perspective, I seemed fine. My brain fog, fatigue, and failing thyroid had no outward signs. Nor was there anything obvious to indicate my aches and pains. I lost significant amounts of hair and gained weight, but because I had a lot of hair and was slender at the outset, few people noticed.

Even as a war rages within your body, many of us can appear completely normal.

The immune system is the coordinator of inflammation. Its primary function is to protect us against pathogens and foreign particles. Pathogens and toxins were major causes of death up until quite recently. Research shows that hunter-gatherers had a longer health span than us (i.e. less chronic disease), but their infant mortality rate (IMR) was much higher at 26-27% due to infections (128; 129; 130). Those with strong, active immune systems had the best chances of survival (131). Though pathogens pose less risk today, we still have the same strong immune systems that kept our ancestors alive. In part, the strength of our immune system is probably what's making so many of us sick with autoimmune and other inflammatory lifestyle diseases in a modern context. It's a well-intentioned, but inappropriate, response to our modern lifestyles.

Your immune system works in two different ways to protect you (132);

1. Via the innate immune response: cuts and bruises, local to the insult. It includes skin and epithelial cells. They form a barrier between the body's cells and the outside world.
2. Via the adaptive immune response. It arises when a system-wide challenge exceeds the abilities of the innate immune response to deal with it.

Both innate and adaptive immune systems can participate in autoimmune disease.

These two systems become active both directly and indirectly through oxidative stress. Once a pathogen is found, innate immune cells will produce reactive oxygen species (ROS). This is a signal to activate inflammatory pathways and to attack the pathogen. Pathogens themselves also cause oxidative stress by producing ROS. This is part of their attack and survival strategy (133). The immune system can detect the pathogen-produced ROS as well. Both sources of oxidative stress boost the immune system and cause inflammation.

Chronic Inflammation: A Departure from Homeostasis

Before we continue, I want to explain a key idea. It is the biological principle of *homeostasis*. Homeostasis is a state where the body's systems work together to function in a certain way (134). A healthy person's immune system maintains this balance. It is there if needed but inactive if not.

In an immunosuppressed person, the body can't fight threats. This can make them very ill. Conversely, a person with chronic inflammation has an immune system in perpetual hyperactivity. It's like a fire engine with all its lights and sirens on. It drives around and around but doesn't put out the fire. Either it can't find it, or it's overwhelmed by the blaze's size. Or the threat it was summoned to combat is not a fire. The challenge is something the immune system isn't equipped to deal with.

Inflammation is a key part of the body's allostatic response. Allostasis is when the body changes to meet a threat. It's doing these things as part of its strategy to return to homeostasis. Oxidative stress has signalled a threat to your immune system, so it has become overactive and needs to act to restore balance.

All autoimmune diseases are inflammatory conditions, and the immune system is key to autoimmune disease. It affects its onset, maintenance, and progression. However, inflammation isn't always bad because we need an inflammatory response in some situations. For instance, exercise causes oxidative stress in the mitochondria. The inflammatory response to this signals the cell to adapt. It does this by making more mitochondria (mitochondrial biogenesis) (135). This is an example of how acute (short-term) inflammation can yield positive adaptations.

In many inflammatory disease conditions, oxidative stress isn't acute; it's chronic. The immune system gets constant messages about oxidative stress in the body. It must stay active to deal with it (136). This sets the backdrop for autoimmune disease to develop.

In autoimmune diseases, chronic oxidative stress continually activates the adaptive immune system. It produces autoantibodies. These differ from regular antibodies. Antibodies are immune cells that identify and neutralise foreign substances like bacteria and viruses. They're antigen-specific, meaning that they recognise and bind to specific molecules on the cell surface of pathogens. Some remain in the body after infection, helping the body remember pathogens it has fought in the past so that it can recognise them more quickly upon re-invasion and mount a speedy response.

Autoantibodies are a type of antibody that fails to distinguish between self and other. They attack the body's tissues and organs (137; 138). The adaptive immune system also triggers a wider inflammatory response to threats. This can sensitise nerves and amplify pain signals. It adds to the perception of aches and pains throughout the body. This can cause widespread musculoskeletal pain and discomfort (139). Though autoantibodies focus on one tissue or organ, autoimmune diseases are a whole-body issue because of the adaptive immune system's systemic effects.

For example, I had Hashimoto's thyroiditis, which causes antibodies to target the thyroid. However, I experienced pain throughout my entire body. Inflammatory molecules were floating around everywhere, not only near the thyroid.

I'm going to run you through a quick overview of how the immune system works below. The body has several ways to sense threats which the immune system must deal with appropriately, calling upon the innate and adaptive systems to deal with them as needed. Let's dive in and go through the process of immune system activation. I've included diagrams to help you understand the immune process.

Let's start with the innate immune system.

The Innate Immune System is Your Firstline Responder

The innate immune system is the body's first defence against infections and oxidative stressors. It works quickly and broadly and includes physical barriers, like skin and mucous membranes. These line your gut and block pathogens from entering the body. Pathogens that breach these barriers should be rapidly intercepted by innate immune cells, which have special pattern recognition receptors (PRRs). PRRs allow them to detect common features of pathogens and mount an appropriate response to them.

One example of a cell with PRRs that's getting a lot of airtime at the moment (for good reasons) is mast cells. Mast cells are a type of white blood cell found throughout the body, especially in exposed tissues. These include the skin, respiratory tract, and digestive system (140). They, along with basophils, another type of innate immune cell, act as sentinels in the various tissues in which they're found (141).

When mast cells are activated, they release substances, including histamines, cytokines, and proteases. Histamines create a conducive environment for other immune cells to travel to the scene of infection, which it does by two main mechanisms. Histamines increase vasodilation, allowing blood to flow more freely. They also increase vascular permeability, which enables immune cells to more readily travel between the bloodstream and the site of activity. Proteases further enable other immune cells to get to the site by breaking down any structures outside cells that might prevent travel. Meanwhile, cytokines attract and activate even more cells to the infection or injury site. This starts the body's initial immune response. This includes calling on cells like macrophages and neutrophils. They can swallow and destroy the invaders. Natural killer (NK) cells also help by finding and killing infected or abnormal cells.

Depending on the context, the complement system, which also forms part of the innate immune system, can also become involved. The complement system is a group of proteins that work together to enhance phagocytosis, trigger inflammation, and destroy pathogens by forming holes in their membranes. The inflammatory environment created by mast cells and basophils acts like a beacon to these and other immune molecules, enhancing the immune response.

The diagram below shows a simplified version of how this works.

The Innate Immune System

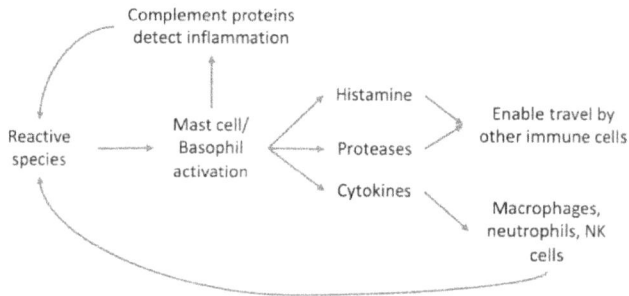

The innate immune system is non-specific, meaning that it doesn't readily distinguish between pathogen types. It mounts a similar response, whatever the source of the incursion. This allows it to be very fast-acting. Information doesn't need to go back to any central network for it to act (142; 143). This is helpful in scenarios where you're best served by a speedy response.

Yet, when a pathogen is more challenging and can't be defeated by the generic mechanisms employed by the innate immune system, a more specific response is needed. This is where the adaptive immune system can help. It has several mechanisms to do so.

For instance, mast cells' influence extends beyond the innate immune system. They can talk to T and B lymphocytes, immune cells that are part of the adaptive immune system. This affects how they work. Mast cells can show antigens to T cells, which helps in specific immune responses. They also release chemicals that can change how T cells develop and work. Also, mast cells can help B cells make antibodies and boost B cells' activity and growth (140).

Mast cells are key mediators of the immune response. They bridge the gap between innate and adaptive systems, helping coordinate and regulate the immune response to threats posed by pathogens, allergens, and damaged tissue.

You may have heard of something called Mast Cell Activation Syndrome (MCAS). This is when mast cells exhibit unchecked activity without any discernible cause. The most well-known MCAS symptoms include flushing, itching, and abdominal pain, often for no apparent reason. You may also experience nasal congestion, flu-like symptoms, diarrhea, constipation, headaches or migraines, and a risk of severe anaphylaxis. MCAS is a key underpinning factor in allergies, though it doesn't directly cause an allergic reaction. It rather just sets the scene for an allergic response. In addition, a wide range of substances can trigger symptoms of MCAS, including some that are non-allergic (144). MCAS can also underpin ongoing upregulation of the adaptive immune system, the mechanisms of which I will describe in the next chapter.

One of the best direct indicators of MCAS is histamine intolerance. Histamine intolerance can occur without MCAS. But it's a good place to start if you have allergic reactions to histamine-rich foods (145). There's a whole world to MCAS and histamine intolerance, including how underpinning genetics interact with environmental factors (including issues with methylation and detoxification pathways) to produce these two often overlapping conditions. Chances are, most of you will have some of the symptoms associated with one or either of them because histamine and mast cells play such an important role in the immune response (146).

Take a look at the diagram below. It highlights symptoms of both histamine intolerance and MCAS. The symptoms in the outer circle are common to both conditions. Those in the inner circle (including autoimmune disease) are specific to MCAS. Which of these can you relate to?

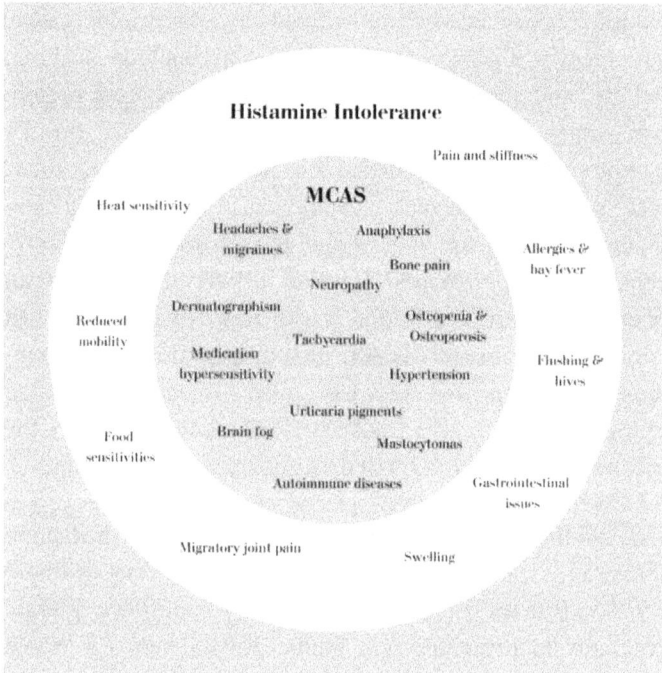

Histamine intolerance and MCAS needed to be treated specially. How to do this effectively varies from person to person. Much of what I discuss throughout this book should alleviate both because it will help you reduce oxidative stress and, therefore, the over-reactiveness of mast cells. Below, I've put a table with some of the most effective compounds to stabilise mast cells. You can take any one of them in isolation (although quercetin and bromelain are best taken together) or take supplements that mix them in smaller doses. You can also try and get these substances from foods. However, I also have a histamine and MCAS protocol on my website, which helps you target them specifically through diet and supplements. If you don't have access to a good practitioner to work with, you may find this useful in calming your innate immune system so that you can more easily work on your adaptive immune system.

Compound	Recommended intake (147)	Food sources (148)
Quercetin + Bromelain (149; 150) *	500-1000mg/day quercetin + 200/400mg/day bromelain	Onions, berries, citrus fruits, apples + pineapple (especially the stem and core)
Liposomal Vitamin C (151)	500–2,000mg/day	Guava, bell peppers, strawberries, broccoli, brussels sprouts, citrus
Luteolin (152)	100-400mg/day	Celery, parsley, chamomile
Turmeric (take with pepper and/or a fat source) (153)	500-2000mg/day	Turmeric

Note that quercetin may not be appropriate if you have ADHD (due to COMT mutations), so it's better to steer clear of it if you have an ADHD diagnosis or know that you have these genetic mutations (154).

The Adaptive Immune System is a Specialist Responder That Malfunctions in Autoimmune Disease

Believe it or not, the majority of your adaptive immune system is housed in your gut. 70-80% of your body's immune cells are found there (155). This makes sense when you think about it. Your gut is the place where pathogens are most likely to enter the bloodstream and, therefore, gain access to your entire body. Having so many immune cells is like having a really good insurance policy for your house when you live in a tropical area. Chances are, you're going to get hit by a cyclone or a tornado sooner or later and need to use it.

The adaptive immune system is highly specific, in contrast to the non-specific innate immune system. Its main function is to identify and eliminate particular pathogens. Lymphocytes, a type of white blood cell, are central to this system. These include T cells and B cells, both of which are produced in bone marrow but migrate to the gut and lymphoid organs once they mature so they can be assigned their respective role.

Different types of T cells have distinct functions. Cytotoxic T cells directly destroy infected cells, helper T cells regulate and support the immune response, while regulatory T cells prevent overactivity in the immune system.

Some B cells become plasma B cells, which produce antibodies. These antibodies bind to antigens, specific molecules on pathogens like viruses and bacteria. These antibodies either mark the pathogens for destruction or neutralise them. This process is essential in defending the body from infections. The cells that produce autoantibodies are plasma B cells.

B cells and sometimes T cells, can also become memory immune cells. Memory cells in the immune system are specialized immune cells that "remember" previous infections or vaccinations. They enable a faster, better response to future exposures. This immunity memory supports the adaptive immune system's ability to fight infections and makes the system precise, specific, and able to remember past infections. These features let it defend the body for life (142).

The problem for people with autoimmune diseases is with their memory immune cells. These can mistakenly recognise the body's own tissues and organs as a threat. They then undergo a process called differentiation, where they change into plasma B cells and start to attack the body's antigens, causing an exaggerated immune response. It may do more harm than good. This is the kind of memory that you want to lose as you get older!

For example, memory cells can identify and react to self-cells. This is due to cross-reactivity. This can happen when your antigens are similar to those of pathogens encountered in the past.

The thing is, your immune system has mechanisms to self-regulate and prevent this kind of issue. It will literally destroy cells that attack you. However, in autoimmune diseases, the cells that regulate memory B cells are impaired. This can happen when DNA methylation isn't working as well as it should. The self-tolerance system breaks down, and they are left unchecked (156). Overactive memory cells are left to run rampant, behaving like someone looking for a fight.

This causes the ongoing production of antibodies and cytokines, which then damage tissues and organs. It can even cause total organ failure (157). Worse, damage to tissues and organs can present more self-antigens to memory cells. It worsens the immune response, and the adaptive immune system then attacks the body even more, promoting a destructive cycle.

Why do these memory cells consistently form to target the self? Why are they on the prowl, looking for something to destroy? And why doesn't the body do more to stop them?

The answer to this is complex and multi-faceted. We've already talked about genetics and issues with their appropriate expression. We're going to talk about lifestyle factors as well. However, it all stems from oxidative stress and mitochondrial dysfunction, causing an ongoing immune response.

Before discussing the causes of oxidative stress and mitochondrial dysfunction, we must understand how the adaptive immune response is maintained. This requires us to take a bit of a deep dive into the nervous system in the next chapter.

Exercise

In the last chapter, we looked at oxidative stress. You assessed your oxidative stress level and how it was affecting you. Now, we're going to take a deep dive into how it's impacting your immune system function. Again, I'm going to ask you to complete a short survey. It will just take a couple of minutes. Keep the results handy so that you can refer back to them later.

Immune System Activity Questionnaire

This questionnaire is designed to help assess whether someone's immune system may be **overactive**, **underactive**, or in **homeostasis**. Please rate each statement on a scale of 1 to 5, where:

1= Strongly Disagree
2 = Disagree
3 = Neutral
4 = Agree
5 = Strongly Agree

Questions:

1. I frequently experience colds, infections, or other illnesses.

2. I feel fatigued even after a full night's rest.

3. I often have digestive issues, such as bloating, constipation, or diarrhoea.

4. I have frequent allergies or allergic reactions (e.g., hives, sneezing, or itching).

5. I experience joint pain or swelling regularly.

6. I often notice hair loss or thinning.

7. I experience anxiety, feel on edge, or have trouble relaxing.

8. My wounds take longer than usual to heal.

9. I have been diagnosed with an autoimmune disorder or experience symptoms like chronic inflammation.

10. I experience hormonal imbalances (e.g., irregular periods, thyroid issues, or changes in appetite).

11. I have a flat or depressed affect (feeling emotionally numb or down).

12. I rarely get sick with bugs or viruses, even when others around me do.

13. I feel that I experience brain fog or trouble concentrating.

14. I often notice skin rashes or eczema flares.

Scoring and Interpretation:

High scores (≥22) on questions 2, 3, 4, 5, 6, 7, 9, 10, 12, 13, and 14 may indicate an **overactive immune system**.

High scores (≥18) on questions 1, 2, 3, 6, 8, 3, 10, 11, and 13 could suggest an **underactive immune system**.

Low scores (generally <3 on each question) indicate that the immune system is likely functioning in **homeostasis**. The absence of major symptoms across these areas suggests a balanced immune response, where the body is neither overreacting nor underreacting to environmental and internal triggers.

Chapter Summary

- The immune system's main role is to protect us from pathogens. Historically, those with the strongest immune systems had the greatest chance of survival.
- There are two main branches of the immune system: the innate and adaptive immune systems.
- These two systems are designed to be upregulated in response to oxidative stress, either produced by pathogens or by the immune system itself as part of its defence system.
- Autoimmune diseases are inflammatory conditions in which the adaptive immune system is chronically upregulated.
- The widespread aches and pains throughout the body commonly experienced in autoimmune diseases are caused by the systemic nature of the adaptive immune system.

- The innate immune system acts as the first line of defence against pathogens, responding quickly but non-specifically to threats.
- The adaptive immune system is slower-acting but is highly specific through its production of B cells and T cells.
- T cells can destroy infected cells, regulate immune responses, and control excess immune activity.
- B cells produce antibodies, proteins that bind to antigen (protein) molecules on pathogens, marking them for destruction or neutralising their harmful effects.
- B cells and sometimes T cells can also develop memory cells, which remember antigens specific to pathogens they've previously encountered.
- Memory cells are advantageous as they can promote a faster response when they re-encounter a pathogen or one similar to it that's previously been encountered but can also mistakenly identify self-made proteins as belonging to pathogens, resulting in autoantibody (self) attacks.
- Normally, problem memory cells are identified and destroyed quickly by the self-tolerance system, but in some instances, such as when DNA methylation is dysregulated, they can persist.
- The damage caused by self-attack can then create further oxidative stress, fuelling immune activity further.

Your Nervous System is Your Body's Master Regulator

"...the body and mind are not separate and we cannot treat one without the other."

Candace Pert, *Molecules of Emotion*

When I was at my sickest, I had especially vivid dreams. Most of these were nightmares, reliving past frightening experiences. The exception was one dream that I had, which was of the ocean near where I grew up. It was a special place for me, somewhere that I'd always experienced a sense of peace and tranquillity. When I was there, every worry or care ceased to exist in my mind.

In the dream, I could always feel the sun on my skin and the wind in my hair. The ocean was a bright, aquamarine blue, cold but so refreshing.

It seemed that the ocean was calling to me, begging me to come home. I resisted for months. One morning, after a vivid dream, I woke up and knew what to do. Within a month, I was back in my home state. But it took me a few more months to work up the courage to move back to my childhood home. Moving home felt so much like failure. Little did I realise that success comes in many different forms.

I still remember the moment I drove up my parents' driveway. The sun was setting, casting a golden glow over the paddock on my right. I wound down my car windows, and the sea breeze came straight in from the east, sending a tingle down my spine. Something shifted within me at that moment. I didn't heal immediately – there was still a lot more work to do – but that moment marked a turning point in my journey.

That moment and what I noticed afterwards got me wondering. Every time I went to the beach and my childhood home, I felt different. How could a setting affect me? Not only was I calmer, but my symptoms subsided as well. I started to get better.

Understanding the Brain-Body Connection

For most of recent history, people saw the brain and body as separate. Many of the systems in the body were also seen as operating separately. But, according to Chrousos (158), modern science is uncovering a relationship between the brain and body.

Whatever happens in one affects what is happening in the other.

Moreover, research shows you feel best when your body systems work together (159). This means having a strong connection between the brain and the body. They are not disparate. They interact and work together to coordinate coherent organism functions. The scientific term for this is "entrainment".

A helpful way of thinking about this might be to think of what the body is. We talk about ourselves and other organisms in their entirety (e.g. me, a cat, a dog) as a non-specific term. It describes the outcome of a system with many parts. As Lynn Margulis and Dorian Sagan (160) described, the whole is important, but you are a multicellular, many-celled organism. The organism is composed of groups of cells that have specific roles (organs. And within those are collections of cells (tissues). And so on. Each cell in the body has its role to play and is motivated by some reason to fulfil it.

What if each cell type had a unique end goal that motivated them? Or do you think that different means should achieve it? Imagine a workplace where everyone has different values and beliefs, which means they have different goals. They might even speak different languages. In any organisation, there will be some variability and diversity. It's inevitable and to be embraced. But if their values, beliefs and goals are vastly different, and they can't even communicate properly to figure things out, it will be difficult to prioritise and make decisions, let alone achieve anything.

In an organism (like you or me), entrainment means all cells and their task systems are aligned. They work well together to achieve a common goal.

Like any good team, your body's cells and collections of cells need a means of communicating with each other. This is the role of the nervous system. It's the master regulator of body operations (161).

What makes it so perfect for this role is its rapid rate of communication. It lets you quickly respond to stressful, dangerous changes in the environment. It's faster at responding to threats than the brain (162; 163). Fast reflexes powered by the nervous system occur in milliseconds, allowing the body to react quickly to threats. Rather than having to think about running away from a lion, your nervous system decides to do this for you.

Normally, your nervous system only undertakes these reflexive reactions occasionally. Your brain does most of the heavy lifting when it comes to deciding how to behave. But if you've faced a lot of situations needing quick reflexes in your life, what do you think might happen? Your nervous system is going to be on the lookout for threats. It expects them. And because of this, you will react more reflexively. The brain will play less of a role in your reactions and behaviours.

This is part of how "muscle memory" works for athletes. When they practice enough, a particular movement becomes instinctive and reflexive rather than something they have to think about.

Instead of acting mostly as a messenger, your nervous system takes charge.

Emotions Underpin Nervous System Activity

I want to give you a quick overview of the mechanics of the nervous system. I think you'll find that the penny will drop here about why the nervous system is so important. You'll also understand why I got so unwell with Hashimoto's when I also had complex post-traumatic stress disorder. It may also give you some insights into the link between your own mental and physical health.

Let's start with neurons. Neurons are the building blocks of the nervous system. They send both chemical and electrical signals, which travel down long projections called axons to reach other neurons, muscles, or glands. Neurotransmitters are small chemical messengers. They are released at synapses, the gaps between neurons, facilitating the transfer of signals. Neurotransmitters act quickly within the nervous system.

Some biochemicals, like neuropeptides, have a broad role in signalling. They act as both neurotransmitters *and* hormones. Their dual nature lets them influence both the nervous and endocrine systems. As neurotransmitters, they cause quick responses (164). As hormones, they have longer-lasting effects (165).

Candace Pert's research in psychoneuroimmunology revealed that neuropeptides form the biological basis for emotions (40; 166). They're made as part of any emotional response, so they help determine how we feel but they also allow the nervous and immune systems communicate. Neuropeptides bind to receptors throughout the body, translating emotional experiences into physiological changes.

Emotions aren't just in the brain. They're whole-body processes.

Neuropeptides essentially link emotional responses with physical health. They don't just influence how you feel from moment to moment. They influence how your entire body operates. This includes the immune system, meaning your emotional state affects your immune system's function via changes in nervous system function.

Your emotional state changes very rapidly in response to changes in your nervous system (164). The nervous system's rapid response to environmental changes can be attributed to its structural properties and the speed of bioelectrical activity. Signalling in the spinal cord, a component of the central nervous system, occurs much faster than in the brain, sometimes at speeds thousands of times greater (162; 163). This rapid reflexivity is an evolutionary adaptation that enables immediate reactions to critical stimuli, such as when faced with a threat.

The nervous system's high reflexivity plays a crucial role in coordinating the functions of other bodily systems. For example, by enhancing the efficiency of your nervous system, you can improve resilience to oxidative stress and bolster your antioxidant defence system. Effective modulation of nervous system function can positively influence other systems, including the adaptive immune system. Ultimately, the nervous system acts as the body's master regulator, orchestrating responses across various physiological systems.

Structure of the Nervous System

The nervous system has two main branches: the central and peripheral nervous systems. The central nervous system consists of the brain and spinal cord. The peripheral nervous system includes all the nerves outside the brain and spinal cord, such as those in your arms, legs, and hands. Without these two systems working together, you couldn't get sensory information from the body (via the peripheral nervous system) to your spine and brain (the central nervous system). Your brain and body would be disconnected. You'd have no conscious experience at all (167).

The nervous system helps you do things you want to do, like going for a walk, cooking a risotto, or finishing a work report. It also controls unconscious things, like breathing, digestion, and your heartbeat.

The autonomic nervous system (ANS) controls the unconscious functions. It spans both the central and peripheral nervous systems. Three main branches comprise the ANS.

· **Sympathetic nervous system (SNS)**

· **Parasympathetic nervous system (PNS)**

· **Enteric nervous system (ENS)**

Many textbooks and scholars bundle the ENS into the PNS. So, they discuss two branches of the ANS. However, it's important to fully understand how the ANS works in the context of autoimmune diseases, so I'm keeping them separate (168).

The SNS is what you can think of as the part of the ANS that induces momentum and movement (169). This isn't all it does, but for the sake of simplicity, we'll think of it like this. One of its primary jobs is to keep our hearts beating. Each time your heart beats, it's because of SNS activity. But, left to its own devices, the SNS would speed up your heart. It would beat at 120 beats per minute at rest, which is too fast (170).

This is where the PNS comes in. A special part of it puts brakes on the heartbeat, keeping your heart rate at approximately 60 beats per minute. If your heart rate is higher than that, it means your SNS is more dominant. If it's lower, then your PNS is slightly more dominant. Either way, these two branches of the ANS should work in concert to regulate your heartbeat and physiology (171). I should note that this isn't all the PNS does. It can also play a role in arousal, though we'll mostly discuss its role in moderating SNS activity here.

The ENS is also important because it regulates gut activity (172). It's in constant communication with the PNS and the SNS. When the PNS is slightly more dominant than the SNS, it signals the ENS to facilitate and oversee digestion. When the PNS withdraws, and SNS activity is dominant, it acts as a signal for digestion to stop. This is how the gut and the brain are connected; it's via the ANS.

Before we go on, it's important to introduce you to the vagus nerve. The vagus nerve isn't actually one nerve; it's a bundle of nerve fibres. They are the main parts of your PNS (173). The terms vagus nerve and PNS are often used interchangeably. For the moment, I'm going to keep things broader and refer to the PNS, but I'll dig into the vagus nerve in more detail shortly.

Polyvagal Theory

As already discussed, the autonomic nervous system (ANS) regulates unconscious bodily functions. It also influences mood and behaviour. Stephen Porges's Polyvagal Theory helps us understand how it's involved social behaviour in mammals, including humans. This theory highlights the vagus nerve's key role in this process (174).

The vagus nerve, or cranial nerve X, is one of the longest and most intricate nerves in the body. It starts in the brainstem and extends through the neck into the thorax and abdomen, innervating various organs and tissues. It has many branches that contribute to regulating different autonomic functions (175).

Porges's work builds on earlier research by Candace Pert and others. It links the ANS's states to specific emotions. Psychologists classify these emotional states as having either a negative or positive valence. This is not to say that they're "good" or "bad." These classifications reflect their impact on brain function and physiological responses (176). As you might be able to imagine, positive valence emotions are things like awe, contentment, wonder, excitement, and love. Negative valence emotions are things like fear, sadness, rage, and despair.

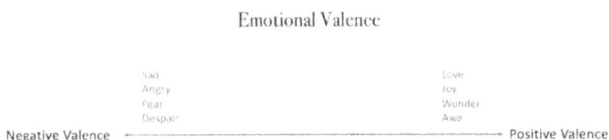

Emotional Valence

Sad		Love
Angry		Joy
Fear		Wonder
Despair		Awe

Negative Valence ⟵————————————————⟶ Positive Valence

Polyvagal Theory splits the vagus nerve into two branches: ventral and dorsal vagal. These, along with the SNS, contribute to the three main states of the ANS in Polyvagal Theory.

Ventral vagal state: Also known as *rest and digest*. It's a state in which the PNS is slightly dominant over the SNS and the ENS is actively facilitating digestion. Our brain and body are in communication with one another. We can do tough mental tasks. We can connect with others. We can feel relaxed but alert. The body and brain are in strong communication with each other. Associated with positive valence emotions.

Sympathetic activation: Also known as *fight or flight*. In this state, our ventral vagus nerve withdraws and the SNS is more dominant. It's a state of mobilisation in reaction to a stressor. The brain's prefrontal cortex shuts down. So, we respond more instinctively to stimuli, rather than rationalising. Associated with negative valence emotions.

Dorsal vagal state: This is known as the *freeze* response. It's a state of paralysis, due to the dominance of the dorsal vagal part of the PNS. Your body is focused on energy conservation, a survival strategy, in the Dorsal vagal state. It usually happens after sympathetic activation fails to create safety. Communication between the brain and body is limited. Our nervous system is more reactive. It's also associated with negative valence emotions.

You can probably guess, from my explanation, how these states relate to some common mental and emotional states (177). Someone in the ventral vagal state would be in a state of generally good mental health. In the sympathetic state, a person likely has more anxiety. The dorsal vagal state can cause feelings of helplessness and low motivation. These are symptoms of depression.

States of the Autonomic Nervous System

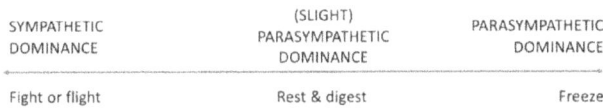

SYMPATHETIC DOMINANCE	(SLIGHT) PARASYMPATHETIC DOMINANCE	PARASYMPATHETIC DOMINANCE
Fight or flight	Rest & digest	Freeze

But the effects of these different states are not limited to your mental health. They are a direct reflection of what's happening for you physically as well. Remember how the ANS coordinates your other bodily systems? When in one particular state for an extended period, it will send a constant signal to those other systems that things in the environment are a certain way. Your immune system will respond accordingly.

Nervous System Coordination of the Adaptive Immune Response

As we've discussed, the immune system has an ideal state of balance, like everything in the body (178). Everyone's immune system is unique. It depends on genetics and lifetime exposure. But in general, you want it primed and ready for action but not active unless there's a threat. When a threat appears, you want it to respond quickly. This will minimise damage from toxins or pathogens. Then, it should return to normal.

The ANS largely coordinates the adaptive immune response. It also restores normal immune function after pathogen and virus infections. Researchers recently found specific neurons in the vagus nerve, at the brainstem's base, that coordinate the adaptive immune response. They experimented on them in mice. When they stimulated these neurons, the mice had a normal immune system. It was ready for action should it be needed but not overactive. However, when these neurons were silenced, the release of inflammatory molecules increased by *300%* (179).

Those with high SNS activity generally have an overactive immune system. Those with high PNS activity generally have a suppressed immune response. One observes optimal immune functioning when the PNS and SNS are in a more balanced state, especially when the PNS *slightly* dominates.

Emotions of negative or positive valence precede each of these states. The immune response can then, in turn, affect emotions. If inflammatory molecules cross the blood-brain barrier, it may trigger a fight-or-flight response. They act as a signal of danger.

Fight or Flight & Immune Activation

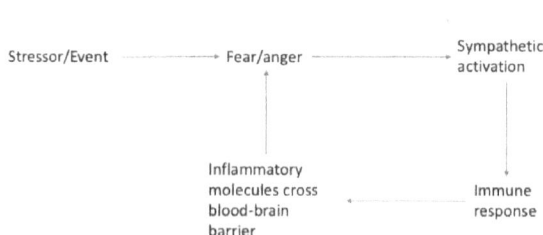

Stressor/Event ·······→ Fear/anger ···········→ Sympathetic activation

Inflammatory molecules cross blood-brain barrier ·········· Immune response

Freeze & Immunosuppression

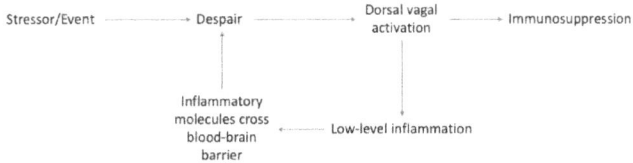

Stressor/Event ········→ Despair ········ Dorsal vagal activation ········→ Immunosuppression

Inflammatory molecules cross blood-brain barrier ←········ Low-level inflammation

In rest and digest, there is no immune activation or suppression. Positive emotions are easily maintained.

Rest & Digest & Immune Resolution

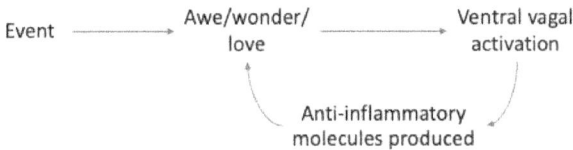

Event ———→ Awe/wonder/ love ——————→ Ventral vagal activation

Anti-inflammatory molecules produced

This aspect of your immune response is now thought to work something like this. When innate immune cells, like mast cells, detect a threat bigger than they can handle, they release signalling molecules. These communicate with the brain. The hypothalamus processes these signals. In response, it upregulates the immune system. This is an unconscious process. It usually causes negative emotions, less vagus and enteric nervous system activity, and a stronger SNS. This higher SNS activity signals the immune system to ramp up, increasing the production of inflammatory molecules (180).

The Adaptive Immune Response

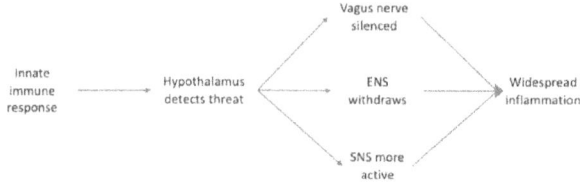

Innate immune response → Hypothalamus detects threat → Vagus nerve silenced / ENS withdraws / SNS more active → Widespread inflammation

Likewise, if the spinal cord gets a threat signal, it can relay this to the brain. This can create negative emotions. These emotions signal the brain, especially the hypothalamus that something is wrong. In response, the hypothalamus signals the vagus nerve to reduce its activity. This shifts the body towards sympathetic dominance and upregulates the immune system (181; 182).

In either case, a greater perceived threat causes a stronger response, both in terms of felt emotions and immune activity.

This works on both ends of the emotional spectrum. We use the term arousal to describe the strength of an emotion. The stronger your emotion, the more intensely you feel it, and thus the more aroused you are.

Remember how we talked about entrainment between all of your body systems earlier? Stronger emotions send a stronger signal to your body's systems to either work well together or to disband their team structure and work separately. The immune system is included in this. High arousal negative emotions signal it to go rogue, either by overactivity or underactivity. High arousal positive emotions signals it to work with your other body systems. It becomes more responsive and adaptive to their needs (183; 184).

High Arousal vs. Low Arousal Emotions

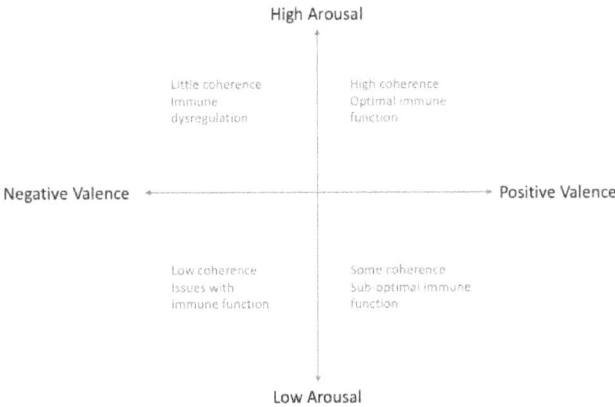

Once the threat has been dealt with, your emotional state changes back to one in the rest and digest spectrum, those emotion states associated with positive valence. Neurons in that same area of the vagus are signalled to come back online. They produce compounds to dampen the immune response. At the same time, the SNS reins in its inflammatory influence (185).

Here's the thing: the adaptive immune system reacts the same to signals from the autonomic nervous system (ANS), no matter the threat. As far as innate immune cells and the hypothalamus are concerned, reactive species are reactive species (RS). Remember how pathogens produce RS as part of their strategy to overwhelm their host? The immune system perceives all RS, even those you produce yourself, as a threat that the immune system needs to deal with. RS we ingest, or that results from pathogens or mitochondrial dysfunction, initiates the same immune response.

Why? Because it's an efficient way to run the system. By upregulating the SNS, we become more immune and behaviourally reactive. This lets us handle many threats at once or a single threat in many different ways. In human evolution, stressful times raise the risk of both injury and infection. This was true during hunts or fights with other tribes.

But it also makes sense in the context of what our immune systems evolved to deal with. Remember how high infant deaths – mostly from pathogens – were in the past? Pathogens have historically been our biggest threat, and they're *still* what your immune system is best adapted to deal with today.

This co-activation of the SNS and immune system explains why mental health issues are common in those with chronic immune dysregulation (186). Both reflect shifts in the autonomic nervous system away from homeostasis, with psychiatric disorders now increasingly seen as largely metabolic disorders. Mitochondrial dysfunction and oxidative stress may cause or worsen them (187).

A key to overcoming autoimmune disease is to teach your nervous system to return to homeostasis. It must receive signals that it's safe to do so, which then lets the immune system know to return to homeostasis (188). We don't want the immune system to be overactive, though we also don't want it to be underactive. That can lead to cancer and other immune issues.

It's worth noting that the nervous system is very reflexive. It goes through different states at different times of the day, sometimes taking only a split second to swap from one state to another. Your immune activity is slower to work than this; it's coordinated by the nervous system's general trend. We consider it overactive or underactive based on that. For example, if the nervous system is more balanced over seven days, even though you might have had moments of rage or fear during that time, your immune system will be less active. This can reduce symptoms and upregulate fewer genes linked to your immune condition.

A flare-up occurs when emotional stress or immune signals trigger a more persistent nervous system shift. This pushes you further along the scale towards sympathetic overactivity, making your immune system more active. As the immune system gears up, it triggers inflammatory genes linked to autoimmune diseases. This creates a storm of inflammation that worsens symptoms. More energy goes to the immune system. This makes you more tired, and you may feel more anxious and irritable.

The nervous system can also undergo wild fluctuations in activity. It can switch from a fierce immune response to an underactive one, causing changes in symptoms and mood. This also increases the risk of cancer or other immunosuppressed conditions.

Having an autoimmune disease likely means you've faced this situation. This is part of the body's allostatic response, an attempt to return to homeostasis.

Thankfully, we know some things that cause dysregulation of the nervous and immune systems, which include both the brain and body. In the next section, we'll go through them. I'll also discuss how to check which affects you most and how to sync your brain and body.

Exercise

You've just learnt how important your nervous system is for regulating immune function. What you're going to do now is figure out how exactly your nervous system is functioning. But to do that, I need to first introduce you to the concept of heart rate variability.

Heart Rate Variability (**HRV**) is a measure of the heart's interbeat intervals. In its most simple form, HRV measures the time difference between beats. More complex calculations of HRV include a measurement of the change in beat-to-beat power output. If you've been told what I was told most of my life, you might think that low HRV is better since the heart is meant to beat steadily, right?

The opposite is true. A healthy heart has a regularly *irregular* heartbeat over a 26-second cycle. It's not a metronome (189). Higher HRV is an indication that your PNS is correctly applying the breaks on the SNS and that there's balance in the ANS. It creates more rest time and lower energy output between beats, but when the heart does beat, there's more action potential, helping to push blood around the body more effectively and bringing all of your bodily systems into a more coherent pattern (190; 191). Your body systems work together more effectively when you have high HRV.

In saying that, there is such a thing as HRV that's too high. This is when the PNS is too dominant. You can experience an increased risk of a range of conditions, including immunosuppression (185). Now that I've overcome my autoimmune disease and am back to doing plenty of exercises, I see this sometimes when I'm doing a little bit too much training in the medium to low-intensity bracket. Because I'm constantly on the go, PNS activity is increased to conserve energy (192). For me, this is often accompanied by a decrease in heart rate to somewhere in the very low 40s.

There's no set number for what your heart rate and HRV should be, and, to be honest, the sweet spot for everyone's heart rate and HRV will likely vary slightly. There are so many different ways of measuring HRV that, unless you have a comparable measurement method, it's very hard to make a recommendation. Mine seems to be around the 46-50bpm (at rest) mark, accompanied by HRV at the highest end of the healthy spectrum. I feel full of energy and clear-headed at this point. But other people may struggle with a heart rate this low and find their immune system is suppressed with the same numbers. This would be denoted by getting sick constantly. I suggest trying to have your resting heart rate (if you can't measure HRV) under 60 and even into the low 50s and your HRV at least in the healthy range for whatever measurement device you're using. This will be a sign that your PNS is slightly more dominant than your SNS, something you almost certainly want to see in autoimmune disease.

So, what's the best way to measure HRV? There are loads of tools out there now – smartwatches, scanners that you can download on your phone and use at different times, plus medical-grade devices. These can all help measure HRV. I have a smartwatch, which I bought to help with marathon training. Most of these devices aren't as accurate as a medical-grade HRV monitor or electrocardiogram, but they can act as good general indicators of what's happening and what throws your HRV out of whack.

The problem is that most smartwatches don't provide moment-by-moment data. With clients, I use something called an emWave Pro, which provides real-time, highly sensitive data on HRV. But for home use, I suggest downloading an app called 'StressScan'. This is not completely accurate, but it can give you a baseline reading to understand what's happening with your nervous system.

Here's what I want you to do:

1. Take a baseline reading of your HRV while at rest and with as few distractions around you as possible. A quiet room is an excellent place to do this exercise. Don't look at the monitor, let your gaze and your thoughts wander. You can also close your eyes if you feel more comfortable. Do this for a minute or so.

2. Now introduce some kind of breathing exercise, such as box breathing (4 counts for breath in, hold 4

counts, 4 counts for exhale, hold 4 counts, repeat) or even simple slow breathing, in for 6 seconds and out for 6 seconds. Maintain this breath rate for approximately two minutes.

Once you've finished, take a look at your HRV device. Do you notice any changes at any specific points in time? How do you feel? In theory, you should see an increase in your HRV at or after the point at which you introduced the breathing practice. If there were any loud noises or distractions, you'll probably notice that they drop your HRV but then if you kept going, you should have recovered back to a higher HRV.

Once you've mastered the breathing technique (this may take a couple of sessions) you can add in one more layer to the process. Go through the first and second steps and then, once your breath has settled in, try to relive your happiest memory or think of your favourite place or a person you love and feel safe with. Imagine whatever place, person, or moment that you decide on in vivid detail, taking care to pay attention to all of the associated sensory information and how whatever you're imagining or remembering makes you feel. Allow that feeling to wash over you. Open up your senses to it.

This is an adapted version of Heartmath's Quick Coherence® technique. I encourage you to have a look at the original version on their website (it will come up if you google it) if you master this easily and want to add in an extra step.

If you struggled with this, then something simple you could try instead is just to look at some pictures that make you feel good. Photos of kittens, nature vistas, your own loved ones – whatever makes you feel either warm and fuzzy or awestruck should help increase your HRV.

Keep track of how your HRV changed during this process by answering the following questions:

1. How much improvement did I see in my HRV in the first two minutes of just breathing?
2. How much did my HRV further improve (or did it go down?!) when I added the memory/visualisation?
3. How easy/hard did this exercise feel?

Keep track of your answers here, as we'll be coming back to them later.

Chapter Summary

*   Historical view saw brain and body as separate; modern science shows they are closely linked.
*   Optimal functioning occurs when body systems work in harmony.
*   Cells and organs should coordinate towards a common goal, akin to a well-functioning team.
*   Nervous system structure comprises neurons and axons; neurons transmit chemical and bioelectrical information, and axons carry electrical signals.

- Neurotransmitters and hormones both communicate within the body, with neurotransmitters acting locally and hormones affecting distant sites.
- Neuropeptides, involved in neurotransmission, link emotions to physiological responses.
- These peptides impact immune function and overall health through emotional states.
- Spinal cord signalling is faster than brain signalling, aiding quick reactions to threats.
- The nervous system's high reflexivity is crucial for coordinating other bodily systems and responding to environmental changes.
- Autonomic nervous system (ANS) includes sympathetic (SNS), parasympathetic (PNS), and enteric (ENS) systems.
- SNS induces movement and increases heart rate; PNS slows heart rate and promotes relaxation; ENS regulates gut activity.
- Polyvagal theory, developed by Stephen Porges, explains social behaviour through the vagus nerve and its branches.
- Three ANS states: ventral vagal (rest and digest), sympathetic activation (fight or flight), and dorsal vagal (freeze response), each associated with emotions.
- The ANS, particularly through the vagus nerve, coordinates adaptive immune responses.
- Stress and immune responses are intertwined; chronic stress can exacerbate immune dysregulation and mental health issues.

- Immune system should be primed but not overactive; dysregulation can lead to autoimmune disease or cancer.
- Nervous system fluctuations can influence immune activity, affecting symptoms and overall health.
- Chronic flare-ups may involve significant fluctuations in nervous and immune system activity.
- Addressing dysregulation involves understanding and managing brain-body interactions and ensuring systems work in sync.

Part 2 – Putting Your Lifestyle Under the Microscope

Causes of Oxidative Stress

"The secret of change is to focus all of your energy not on fighting the old, but on building the new."

Socrates

Before I was diagnosed with Hashimoto's, I was so confused. In the past, I had success in resolving health issues through diet and exercise. These no longer worked. I had to completely change tactics to get the kind of response I was looking for.

This meant making many changes. I revised my approach and reassessed my fundamental self-perception and worldview. I began to realise that many things I thought were true were a version of the truth I had constructed.

This is something we all do throughout our entire lives, especially when we're younger. When you're young, you're naïve and open to new ideas. But you can learn more as an adult, too. Your brain and body are wired to learn. They absorb new information and make sense of it. However, unless challenged, they can then create persistent patterns of thought and behaviour.

This is a valuable feature of human development. High plasticity early in life lets you adapt to different situations and circumstances you find yourself in. Yuval Noah Harari, author of *Sapiens,* points out that it's likely the main reason for humans' success in many environments (193). Our adaptive brains let us change our behaviours to fit our settings.

A loss of plasticity as we age is also a valuable adaptive mechanism. Knowledge is created through a cumulative process. You make sense of your current experience based on your past. It's a mix of what has happened and what you've learned.

But as you age, your ideas about the world become more fixed. With more experience, you have more to draw on. Gene expression changes also occur. They decrease your brain's ability to learn new things. If you think back to what I mentioned in the genetic section about critical periods in Chapter One, this will make sense.

For example, early childhood, from birth to age two, is a time of rapid brain growth and plasticity. The visual cortex's synaptic density peaks at six months. It then undergoes pruning, reflecting the brain's adaptation to visual experiences (194). This critical period is vital for developing sensory and cognitive functions. Experiences then shape the brain's structure and function.

Once you reach the age of around 25, your brain becomes less plastic. Doing some things on autopilot is a result that allows you to do bigger tasks. Goals such as progressing your career or caring and providing for children become more of a priority. Many skills you learned in childhood help you do these things without feeling overwhelmed. You wouldn't get very far in the world if you spent every morning learning to re-tie your shoelaces.

What this means is that how you think and what you do later in life are built on skills that you've learnt early in life. It's tough to be happy and healthy as an adult if your childhood beliefs and behaviours are based on false ideas or misperceptions.

This is what I discovered when I was trying to make sense of what was happening to me. I had to unpack all I knew about myself. I had to sort through it, discard what no longer fit, and repack some ideas to make more sense of what I was learning. It was a painful and exhausting process, but it was also the most worthwhile process I've ever done for myself. I began to understand why I had adopted certain behaviours in the past. In doing so, I realised what once made sense now seemed illogical and unhelpful.

I also recognised that I had sheltered myself from some past events. At the time, doing that kept me safe from hopelessness and despair. But now, it was part of what was making me sick. It didn't just cause me emotional turmoil. My beliefs shaped my daily behaviour. And those behaviours were making me sick.

Fortunately, though your brain plasticity declines as you age, you never lose the ability to learn new things and reshape your behaviour. Learning is lifelong. We know this from studies on ageing and learning (195). You can adopt habits that will support your health for life.

I'm sure that by now, you're wondering what exactly causes oxidative stress and what you can do about it. You may even have some ideas based on what I've shared already.

This section investigates the root origins of oxidative stress. You must understand, though, that autoimmune diseases are lifestyle diseases. There isn't one "cure" for autoimmune disease because it's not caused by one thing. It's caused by many things.

As discussed in the introduction, we know that if autoimmune diseases were heritable only, the prevalence rate would be constant. Yet, incidence and prevalence rates are rising, especially in recent decades. Because they often co-occur with other non-heritable conditions, they can largely be attributed to the environmental influences of lifestyle.

Many things in our lifestyles cause inflammation. They fall into five main categories. Mental and emotional well-being, diet, environmental toxins (chemicals and inorganic compounds, viruses, and bacteria), sleep, and physical stressors (like over or under-exercising). I call these the foundations of Ecological Nutrition. This concept outlines how external nourishment can enhance genetic expression, creating internal well-being.

I'll discuss each of the five causes in detail on the following pages. These causes operate together, not in isolation. They're cumulative. At the local level, the inflammatory molecules released to deal with them are specific and perform different roles. However, when multiple immune pathways are activated concurrently, the overall inflammatory impact may amplify in a way that appears less discriminating. Their combined effect is proinflammatory, meaning that they all contribute to a response from the immune system. In addition, their combined effects can be nonlinear. The immune system's reaction isn't necessarily proportionate to the amount of oxidative stress but can be exponential (196).

In saying this, not all of these will necessarily be contributing to your condition. It depends on your unique circumstances and lifestyle.

As we go through each of these, I encourage you to assess your daily habits and practices in light of what I share. What have you been doing in the past that may have been acting as the trigger that set your immune system off? What beliefs underpin those behaviours? What's in your power to change? And what do you need to let go of because it no longer serves you?

How Your Body Keeps the Score at a Cellular Level

"The best way out is always through."

Robert Frost

I had serious issues with my mental health before I developed Hashimoto's thyroiditis. For a couple of years, I yo-yoed between states of extreme anxiety and depression. Then, several compounding traumatic events made my mental health take an even worse turn. I developed complex post-traumatic stress disorder (CPTSD). Aside from the panic attacks and nightmares, one of my most prominent symptoms was a strong sense of dislocation, not only from others but also from myself. This is a typical symptom of trauma (197). When we can't control what's happening around us or within us, we withdraw. It's like an inbuilt safety feature to protect us from physical and emotional pain.

I began journaling a year or so after I developed CPTSD, on my Mum's recommendation. I resisted initially, as we often do when advice comes from family. But once I finally tried it, I found that words flowed out of me like water. Some days, I spent hours journaling.

I discovered through this process that past events had affected me profoundly. As I began writing about them, I realised how lonely I had been throughout most of my childhood. I hadn't felt a sense of belonging in the community that we moved to when I was eight. I also understood that being bullied by a teacher in primary school had made me feel powerless. Being mocked and shamed by someone I wasn't allowed to argue with shook my confidence. It also started a pattern that has taken years to break.

I stopped standing up for myself. My grades slipped. I withdrew and ceased answering in class. My sole purpose when I left the house each morning was to become invisible.

When I was bullied by two girls only a year or two older than me in my first year of high school, I was at a loss. The experience with my primary school teacher taught me the safest thing to do was avoid my problems. For nearly a year, I sat as far away from them as possible on the bus, cringing in my seat. I was waiting to have insults or spit balls - or both - hurled at me. During lunch and recess, I kept my guard up in the hallways. I found myself pushed to the concrete floor from behind on more than one occasion. Every day was more and more terrifying. The situation was only resolved when my brother told my Mum, who told the deputy principal at the school. I still remember the day he confronted them when the bus was pulling into school and feeling both confused and relieved when they followed him to his office. Yet, while the bullying stopped, I was still afraid. I thought I didn't have the power or authority to take care of myself.

A miserable few years ensued. When I was 14, and men started to pay unwanted attention to me, I reacted in the same way. I froze and kept silent, hoping that they would go away.

This story doesn't end well. I'll spare you the details, but maybe it's no wonder that my first long-term relationship was with someone jealous, possessive, and violent towards anyone who threatened me. Eventually, it turned into a nightmare of coercive control and passive aggression towards me. He made me feel safe until he didn't.

It was a relief when my next relationship was with someone who didn't want too much commitment. Except then he took me to court and denied ever having had an intimate relationship with me.

These pendulum swings characterised so much of my life up until recently. I went from one extreme to the other. From being the chattiest, most inquisitive student to the quietest. From the child who would challenge anything that seemed unjust or untrue to the teenager who didn't know how to say no. From being with a boyfriend who wouldn't leave me alone once we broke up to a boyfriend who denied my very existence.

All this and more made sense once I began journalling. It was like having a timeline of my life written out. For years, I had buried my pain in a dark place inside me. I was afraid to let it into the light. But as I wrote, I realised that burying it hadn't made it go away. It had turned ordinary pain into lifelong suffering. It was like a wound festering under a bandage that was never washed and re-dressed and given air to breathe.

At some point, I came upon the realisation that the only way out of suffering is through it. I had to relive my past traumas, bring them out into the open air, understand them, and finally allow myself to be free.

The Impacts of Trauma

At this point, it's probably worth briefly explaining what trauma is. We hear the term a lot nowadays. It's important to have some context to understand what's meant when we talk about it.

Everyone experiences some kind of traumatic event within their lifetime. This includes predictable events like a grandparent dying or the loss of a beloved pet. Less predictable events like a car crash or being bullied at school can also be included. Yet not everyone is traumatised by these events. It's normal to feel some sadness in response to death or frightened by a car crash. But, when events stay with you, you are said to be traumatised. You relive them in your mind and, often unconsciously, in your behaviours.

According to Dr. Peter Levine, you relive these events because they disempowered you (198). Because you haven't been able to appropriately respond to the situation, your body and mind become trapped in limbo. You try to replay the traumatic events to find a loophole, constantly searching for a way to step in and change the outcome. It's a bigger, all-consuming version of ruminating. You know when you can't move past something that happened? It might be something smaller, like a mistake at work. You play different scenarios out in your mind, wondering if you could have altered the result, thinking *if only I'd done or said something different.*

Trauma is when this happens on a continual basis, even without you knowing that you're doing it. But as we all know, you can't change the past. Yet, even though it's a pointless exercise, you circle the same story, trapped by it.

Trauma can show up in many ways. Psychiatric conditions can be linked to childhood trauma (199; 200; 201). This includes conditions like attention deficit hyperactivity disorder (ADHD), schizoaffective disorder, and borderline personality disorder. Though genetic factors can create a predisposition to them, many experts now view psychiatric conditions as mainly caused by childhood trauma. Their development is context-dependent.

These conditions are seen as a result of changes to neurocircuitry. They alter behaviour, helping a child's chances of survival by acting as adaptations that serve those who develop them, at least at first. But for us as adults, they become maladaptive. Our environment and social circumstances have changed. Perhaps you had a wonderful upbringing, surrounded by loving family and friends. If not, you are hopefully in a much safer place as an adult than you were in your early life. The challenge for those of us who grow up without a sense of safety and those working in the trauma field is to encourage the brain to abandon its old circuitry. We need to establish new, more appropriate behaviours (202; 203).

Because of these trauma-induced changes in neurocircuitry, people with psychiatric disorders often struggle to create a routine that supports a healthy redox balance. Their sympathetic nervous system is more active due to reliving traumatic experiences, resulting in hyper-arousal. And their emotions are sending a constant signal to their immune system: attack! Because of this, there's a tendency for those with psychiatric conditions to have elevated inflammation biomarkers (204; 205).

Researchers have studied the link between stress and inflammation for over 30 years. The first strong evidence of a link between the immune system and emotional stress came from the Adverse Childhood Events (ACEs) study in the late 1990s. These studies used a questionnaire listing possible childhood adverse events. It asked participants to tick those they had experienced.

The questionnaire included events like:

- physical and verbal abuse

- parental divorce

- sexual assault

- household conflict.

The earliest study linked the questionnaire results to outcomes. These included pharmacy use, emergency room visits, and mortality. The study found that higher ACE scores were linked to worse health outcomes (206). Later, the ACEs questionnaires were re-administered to a different group of participants. They compared their results to some health outcomes, including immune function. The researchers found that people who had two or more of these events were between 70% and 100% more likely to be diagnosed with one of three autoimmune disorder groupings as identified through their hospital records (207).

Recent research has studied the link between post-traumatic stress disorder (PTSD) in war veterans and autoimmune disease. Vets with PTSD were *58% more likely* to get an autoimmune disease within five years than their peers without PTSD (208). Parallel findings are also now emerging around CPTSD. CPTSD is similar to PTSD in how it presents, though it is often linked to many compounding events that cause long-term emotional stress (209).

Research has confirmed that the brains of people under stress or trauma produce inflammation. The release of adrenaline and noradrenaline causes this. The autonomic nervous system (ANS) then receives a signal that something's up. It starts gearing up the immune system by activating the sympathetic nervous system (SNS). Once the perceived threat has been dealt with, the parasympathetic nervous system (PNS) comes online, with the vagus nerve playing a leading role in the resolution of inflammation.

It does this through a series of complex mechanisms as part of what's known as "the inflammatory reflex" (185). Though developed by a different researcher, Kevin Tracey, the steps that take place in the inflammatory reflex help explain how Stephen Porges' Polyvagal Theory relates to immune function. At a cellular level, what happens is that the balance of electrolytes changes, inducing a widespread change in cellular activity throughout the body to mobilise resources for fight or flight.

Glucocorticoids, a class of hormones, are then released. The most well-known of these is cortisol. It has two main jobs. One is to moderate the inflammatory response and the other is to maintain resource mobilisation. We'll take a closer look at cortisol in just a moment but this this why chronically elevated cortisol is seen as problematic: because it allows us to stay in a state of fight or flight *and* immune activation for extended periods of time, creating oxidative stress.

This doesn't necessarily *only* happen at the time of the event. Constant activation of the SNS and the inflammatory reflex can cause changes in physiology and brain function that are ongoing. For instance, the locus coeruleus (LC) is part of the brain. It stores short-term memories of the day's most emotional events. During the rapid eye movement (REM) sleep of a non-traumatised person, the LC deactivates via a reduction in SNS activity and increased PNS activity. This lets memories move elsewhere in the brain to become long-term. It wipes the LC clean for new memories to be gathered and processed the next day (210). In people with PTSD and trauma, this process doesn't happen because the nervous system doesn't follow its natural circadian rhythm. So, traumatic events are remembered vividly, as if they are from the present, with an accompanying nervous system state. This can last for months or even years (211). In many instances, this vivid remembering will be accompanied by cellular changes associated with the inflammatory reflex, as well as cortisol release. The final step of inflammation resolution doesn't take place because as far as the nervous and immune systems are concerned, you're still under attack (212).

What this means is that a strong, well-regulated vagus nerve helps you sleep better. It also helps your brain forget the past and form new memories.

The brain and body are in constant communication. They create a feedback loop via the SNS and PNS. Chronic mental and emotional stress, or a severe stressor, can activate the feedback loop. The body and brain feed into each other, causing a constant inflammatory response.

How Cortisol Causes Oxidative Stress

Let's put all this into the context of oxidative stress and changes in your redox balance by looking at the glucocorticoid cortisol. Glucocorticoids are steroid hormones that regulate various processes in the body, including stress. Cortisol plays a key role in this system. Earlier, I mentioned that cortisol can be an oxidative stressor. I'm now going to explain why.

Before we jump in, I want to emphasise that cortisol is important to how your body functions. Cortisol is not bad in and of itself. It plays key roles in the brain and body, especially during acute stress, but also in regulating metabolism and the sleep-wake cycle. It's normal and healthy to produce some cortisol at specific times of the day or in response to certain stimuli. Prednisone, which is sometimes prescribed for people with autoimmune diseases, is a drug that has anti-inflammatory effects because it mimics cortisol (213). As I've already mentioned, cortisol itself can be anti-inflammatory. Released in the right quantities, at the right time of day, it's anti-inflammatory (214). When it becomes problematic, mental and emotional stress becomes chronic. Chronic stress disrupts cortisol production's natural cycle.

There are several ways that cortisol acts as an oxidative stressor. But the main way is, of course, by causing mitochondrial dysfunction. Cortisol exposure interferes with how cells generate and recycle mitochondria.

For example, cortisol disrupts the balance of mitochondrial fission. This is the process where one mitochondrion divides into two during cell division. Cell division is how your body makes new cells. It helps grow a tissue or organ or replace old, worn-out cells. Proper distribution of mitochondria between cells is crucial for effective energy production (215).

Similarly, cortisol influences a process known as mitochondrial fusion. As you can guess from the name, it means mitochondria are fusing. Mitochondria do this to protect their DNA, which is separate from the cell nucleus. It contains the instructions they use for energy production and other functions. For example, fusion is needed to fix damage to their DNA. Mitochondrial DNA sustains damage when fusion fails to occur successfully, and mitochondria become less effective at their jobs (215).

Cortisol production is meant to be a short-term, adaptive response. It ensures energy is ready for "fight or flight" in a SNS-dominant state. The moment a cell runs out of glucose for quick energy, there's plenty more ready to replenish it.

However, chronic high cortisol causes problems. It raises blood glucose, leading to insulin resistance. Insulin is essential for shuttling glucose into cells as it acts like an escort for glucose. With insulin resistance, cells refuse insulin. They have enough glucose. So, they reduce insulin entry points which raises your fasting blood sugar. The glucose your cells deny entry to stays in your bloodstream (216).

The first problem is that this then leads to a rise in something called the polyol pathway. It becomes more active in an attempt to deal with all the extra sugar. To start the polyol pathway, an enzyme called nicotinamide adenine dinucleotide phosphate (NADPH) is needed. NADPH helps make glutathione (GSH). It's your body's most important antioxidant (217). If the NADPH gets used in the polyol pathway, there's not much left to make GSH and your antioxidant defence system weakens.

The second problem is that another molecule, nicotinamide adenine dinucleotide (hydride) (NADH), is produced as a by-product of the polyol pathway. NADH is NADPH with the phosphate removed. It can then alter energy production and increase metabolic ROS generation (218). So, it ends up being a double whammy. Not only is the antioxidant defence system compromised but there are also more ROS to deal with.

But it's not only GSH production that's impaired by cortisol production. Cortisol can also affect enzymes, other than NADPH. These enzymes, including superoxide dismutase, catalase, and glutathione peroxidase, produce antioxidants. This can cause further oxidative stress (219).

Cortisol also influences the immune system through direct action. An acute cortisol response can downregulate the immune system by repressing the activity of T and B-cells, as well as by stabilising mast cells. It's an adaptive response to stress, meant to temper the inflammatory reflex and stop it from damaging your own cells and tissues. However, chronic cortisol exposure *desensitizes* immune cells to its effects. It can no longer dampen their response, leading to the over-production of pro-inflammatory cytokines like Tumour Necrosis Factor-alpha (TNF-α), Interleukin-6 (IL-6), and Interleukin-1 beta (IL-1β). Antibody production can also be increased. These inflammatory molecules kill pathogens by releasing ROS that damage invading viruses and bacteria. But when there are no viruses or bacteria present, they do damage to your own body instead (220; 221).

Oxidative stress in the brain can also result from too much cortisol. It may worsen any existing mental or emotional stress by increasing glutamate release. Glutamate is the brain's main excitatory neurotransmitter. It does exactly what it sounds like – it makes the brain more active and excitable.

Glutamate facilitates things like learning, memory, cognition, and brain development (222). It's important to have enough, or you can feel sluggish and tired. You may also get "brain fog." But when we have too much glutamate, a condition known as excitotoxicity can develop. Excitotoxicity can damage or kill neurons in the brain. Excitotoxicity is tightly linked with mental health conditions such as depression and PTSD. At a cellular level, too much glutamate can overstimulate N-methyl-D-aspartate (NMDA) receptors. They are key to forming memories. This overstimulation increases the production of RS and can eventually impair and destroy parts of the hippocampus, a brain area that plays a major role in memory and learning. This results in memory and learning deficits in people with various psychiatric conditions (223).

I've laid out these effects of chronically excess cortisol in the diagram below.

Cortisol and Inflammation

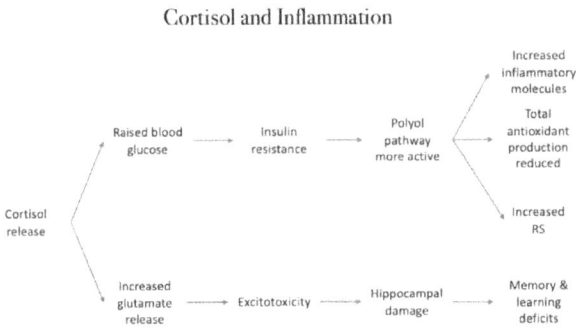

It's important to note that these mechanisms can affect mitochondrial DNA and its expression. They can cause oxidative stress and increase ROS, which harms mitochondrial DNA. Oxidative stress can also damage enzymes that repair DNA (224).

Stress harms you at the cellular level.

Traumatic Stress and Behaviour

Mental and emotional stress doesn't only affect us at the cellular and physiological levels, though. It's often accompanied by behavioural changes.

Remember the ACE study? The lead researcher in the first study was Vincent Felitti. While working at an obesity clinic, he noticed that many patients were dropping out of the program he ran. You might think it would be the patients who struggled most with weight loss and weren't seeing results. Actually, the opposite was true.

Many of the dropouts were *successfully* losing weight. What became clear upon further investigation was that "obesity was not their problem; their obesity had become their protective *solution*" to the problems they had experienced in early childhood (225). Being overweight or obese helped these people hide themselves from perpetrators. They saw it as a safety mechanism. One female study participant hinted that being overweight reduces the likelihood of being raped. Male participants feared weight loss because it made them vulnerable to violence as they no longer had an intimidating figure.

Vincent Felitti faced scepticism when he presented his findings at a 1990 conference, years before the first ACEs study was published. Yet, by the time I'm writing this book in 2024, the first ACEs paper published in 1998 has had over 22,000 citations. In the world of academic literature, that's a staggering amount of people referencing your work. The initial ACEs study is, without question, one of the most influential publications of the last thirty years. It laid the foundations for today's research into trauma and its long-term health effects.

We now know that acute and chronic stress, including trauma, can impact people in many ways, especially if experienced in childhood. This is likely because children are more plastic in their thinking. Their beliefs, values, and attitudes are still forming. They're like a blank canvas ready for someone to make an impression. Those early brushstrokes form a backdrop for how the rest of the painting will turn out. But they are also more likely to be traumatised. They have less control over themselves and those around them.

As you now know, this can have lasting (but not irreversible!) effects on the brain and body, as well as behaviour. One reason for its profound impact is that it shapes your adult behaviour. Addictions are an example of this. Addictions are seen as a way for traumatised people to get the biochemical pleasure of close, intimate relationships. For the traumatised person, intimacy often doesn't feel safe. Yet connection is something we all crave. Those who can't find it in social interactions must seek other ways to feel safe and connected.

A strong, consistent hit of a neurotransmitter brings a rush. But over time, it makes your brain's neuroreceptors less sensitive to it, so you need more and more to get the same high. You'll do anything to activate those neuroreceptors. This includes addictive behaviours like over-exercising, binge eating, and overworking. The conventional view of addiction is changing. It's not *just* about substance abuse. It also includes the harmful, excessive use of any behaviour or substance to get the neurotransmitter hit (226; 227).

Let me give you an example of this from my own life. My teacher bullied me, and then other students also bullied me, which made me feel like I didn't belong. I hated school. So, I started eating all the sugary foods I could find at the school canteen. I put on unhealthy weight, but for a short time, while I was eating them, I felt much better about being there. Afterwards, I felt terrible because of the physiological impacts of eating those foods, but also the psychological impacts of weight gain in a society obsessed with stick-thin female bodies. So, two years after whipping up that obsession, I developed an eating disorder. I became addicted to the rush and that came with witnessing my weight loss. I felt a sense of control I'd unknowingly been craving. A few years later, I became obsessed with exercise. I also abused alcohol in my late teens and devoted myself to work in my late twenties.

I felt temporarily better when I pushed myself in these ways. They distracted me from my anxious thoughts and changed my brain and body chemistry.

Once I faced my feelings from when I was being belittled by my teacher in class, things began to change. It wasn't an overnight process. It took time for me to unravel. But once I did, I was able to let go of my addictive behaviours and adopt new, healthier ones.

I took exercising, eating healthily, drinking, and working to extremes. While some of these behaviours might normally be considered healthy, the extremes to which I did them made them *unhealthy*. Though I never became addicted to an illegal substance, my obsessions affected my daily life. They changed my relationship with myself and others, and caused oxidative stress that hurt my health and damaged my immune system.

As we end this chapter, I urge you to consider: what past events, whether one or many, may have eroded your sense of safety and well-being? And what habits or obsessions might you have developed to control your environment?

The sooner you can understand and address these things, the sooner you'll start feeling better. Ignoring emotional stress and trauma won't make them go away.

On a personal note, I tried many, many things early on in my journey with autoimmune disease to heal myself. None of them worked until I had begun to successfully address my mental health issues. This wasn't enough on its own to put me into remission on its own, but it was the catalyst that sparked my healing journey.

It's also why I went back to university to study mental health. I wanted to help people with both mental health issues and chronic diseases. If you don't feel good about yourself, the knowledge and tools to change your behaviour are irrelevant. You won't be motivated to implement any of what you learn.

Though knowledge is indeed power, we shouldn't overstate its importance. It acts as the fuel for change. Emotions are the engine. They drive you to want to make your life better, using knowledge to strategise and decide how to do it (228). You must face past hurts, learn from them, and change your ways. Only then can you embrace a healthier, happier future.

Exercise

Create a timeline of significant life events, behaviours, and health concerns. You've just heard how powerful journalling was for me. The reason why is that it laid out specific events in my life and made me understand how they were connected to my behaviours. I did this inadvertently. By doing this exercise, you'll do it in a much more direct way.

You don't need to do it as a journal, though you can if that's your preference. You can do it as a visual timeline on a continuum, you can do it as an artwork, or you could even do it as a form of interpretative dance.

Whatever helps you make sense of your memories is the right approach.

Just make sure you have some way of coming back to it later because it's going to be an important tool for you to use.

Use the following prompts if you need to. These are inspired by the Power Threat Meaning Framework, which has been proposed as a new way of understanding the role of environmental factors in mental health (229). You can use the prompts to inform how you create the timeline around each life event.

I recommend starting with your earliest life events first, then moving chronologically along your timeline. It will be easier to make sense of your life this way. If you're in therapy, this may also be something you could do with your therapist.

1. What has happened to you? *When do you remember feeling unsafe or ill at ease?*
2. How did it affect you? *What emotions did you experience? Were you afraid, anxious, depressed, helpless, or angry?*
3. What sense did you make of it? *What was the story you told yourself about what happened? What beliefs arose from that incident or incidents?*
4. What did you have to do to survive? *How did your beliefs about what happened shape your behaviour? How did you change as a person?*

Chapter Summary

- Trauma can be defined as an event or series of events that are experienced as disempowering and are relived over and over (often unconsciously) through thoughts and behaviours.
- Many psychiatric conditions are now attributed to trauma.
- Trauma can lead to not only behaviours that may increase oxidative stress but also increase inflammatory biomarkers as a result of persistent (but not permanent) changes in physiology and brain function, such as how your memory works.
- The more exposure we have to emotional stress and trauma, the more likely we are to experience immune system dysregulation.
- When the inflammatory reflex is initiated, the PNS withdraws, and the SNS becomes more active.
- While cortisol plays important and useful roles in the body, it can lead to mitochondrial dysfunction when produced in high amounts by interrupting processes known as fission and fusion.
- Cortisol can also increase insulin resistance through a process known as gluconeogenesis, where it turns non-carbohydrate fuel sources into glucose.
- It can also disrupt processes involved in the synthesis of antioxidants, including glutathione, your body's master antioxidant, while simultaneously increasing ROS.
- Chronic cortisol exposure can lead to the overproduction of inflammatory molecules within the immune system.

- Cortisol can lead to the over-production of a neurotransmitter called glutamate, leading to brain cell death and deficits in learning and attention.
- Research shows that mental and emotional stress also induces behavioural changes, some with serious health consequences, including addictions, especially when we're subject to stress early on in life.

Food is More Than Just Sustenance

"What most people don't realise is that food is not just calories; it's information. It contains messages that connect to every cell in the body."

Dr. Mark Hyman

Food can be either a source of nourishment or detrimental to your health. Yet, no other health topic has been so misinformed and controversial. This section is about breaking through all the 'food noise' so that you can decide what to believe and what to ignore.

Many dietary factors contribute to oxidative stress. I'm going to discuss the most important ones. I'm not going to tell you exactly what to eat, though, as I'm a proponent of personalised nutrition, plus, there will be a little bit more information on personalised nutrition in section three.

The truth is, what you need is likely different than what I need. It's based on your biology, context, goals, and your autoimmune journey. I want to provide you with information to help guide you about what to eat based on your needs. At the same time, I want to leave some wiggle room for personalisation based on your goals, preferences, and genetics.

One of the simplest ways to tailor your diet to your needs is to check how food affects you. Pay attention to how you feel for a few hours after a meal. Then, adjust your food intake based on that. That said, small intestinal bacterial overgrowth (SIBO) and mould exposure can impact what you have an appetite for. We'll discuss these in another chapter but notice if you often feel unwell after eating foods that theoretically should be good for your health. How you feel is an important clue that can guide you towards making better choices for you *personally.*

The Enteric Nervous System, Stress, & Diet

Before we discuss diet, I want to connect stress and diet to what you've learned about the nervous system and mental health. Mental and emotional stress affects the gut through its links to the autonomic nervous system (ANS). Remember the enteric nervous system (ENS), the third branch of the ANS? The ENS is a vast network of 400-600 million neurons of up to 20 types. They are located along the inner wall of the digestive tract (230). Its role is to manage digestion.

The ENS can act largely independently, so it is often called the "second brain." It stays in close communication with the sympathetic nervous system (SNS) and the parasympathetic nervous system (PNS). When glucocorticoids in the brain signal it's time to go to war, they ramp up the immune system. The immune system receives that message via changes in vagus nerve activity and increased sympathetic dominance. In response, the ENS and gut microbiota release neuropeptides and neurotransmitters and these substances upregulate the immune system. Remember how 80% of the immune system is housed in the gut and T and B cells are assigned their functions there? At a local level, this allows the ENS to modulate the immune response within its direct vicinity. But because so much of the immune system is housed in the gut, it has implications for your entire body.

It's why some people experience brain fog, fatigue, and irritability at the same time they experience stomach pain and bloating. What they're experiencing isn't just happening in their gut, but affects immune and nervous system function in their entire body.

The withdrawal of the ENS under sympathetic activation also opens up little cells in the small intestine lining called tight junctions. In a healthy person, tight junctions *selectively* allow nutrients to pass through the gut wall into the bloodstream, with the ENS regulating their activity. They then transport the nutrients to where they're needed. The problem is when the immune system is on high alert, they tend to be open all the time. This lets anything that fits through them into the bloodstream (231). Now, the body can't eliminate toxins and waste as easily, but it does make food more readily available to muscles and other tissues if they need it for a fast response to a threat. These molecules can then circulate in the bloodstream - not only food but dangerous toxins, bacteria, and even viruses.

In the short term, this might be useful because it increases food availability so your cells can make energy more quickly. But in the long term, it can cause chronic inflammation (232). This is what's thought to be happening in leaky gut syndrome.

Wheat and its relatives, rye and barley, have a gluten protein called gliadin, which can break through the small intestines' tight junctions and circulate in the bloodstream. For this reason, gluten has been linked to many chronic health issues. They include nutritional deficiencies, osteoporosis, infertility, some cancers, and autoimmune diseases (233; 234; 235). Many holistic practitioners ask clients to avoid gluten due to its effects on tight junctions.

Some of you will be able to get around the gluten problem by eating sourdough bread. Its gluten is mostly broken down, especially in those fermented longer and slower (236). The longer, the better.

Some big commercial chains and supermarkets sell "sourdough." These are not suitable as they often have short fermentation times. They only add a bit of sourdough culture plus some commercial yeast. This is why they can be called "sourdough". It also lets manufacturers make them quickly and cheaply. However, there's a high risk they might hurt your gut health as the gluten has not been broken down enough. Source authentic sourdough from an artisan baker and ask how long it has been fermented.

That said, if you still react (bloating, nausea, low energy) after consuming it, then please avoid it. Be aware that if you want to reintroduce sourdough or anything else you are sensitive to, you may need to re-familiarize your immune system, as allergies can develop when you stop eating certain things with a high inflammatory response (237). This should go without saying, but for those with anaphylaxis, if you ever reintroduce anything you're allergic to, please do this under the guidance of an appropriate health professional.

Processed Foods Are a Giant No

While we're on the topic of foods to limit or remove from your diet, let's discuss processed foods. Processed foods are packaged items with multiple ingredients. Some processed foods, like natural yogurts and sourdough bread, have only a few natural ingredients. You would find these in nature. What I mean when I say processed foods are those with various additives and laboratory-synthesized ingredients not found in nature.

Processed foods contribute to oxidative stress through several mechanisms. Firstly, they often have high levels of unhealthy vegetable and seed oil fats, like trans and oxidised fats. Excessive consumption can increase reactive oxygen species (ROS) in the body (238). Secondly, added sugars in processed foods can cause glycation. This is where sugars react with proteins and lipids to generate ROS and promote oxidative stress (239).

Also, processed foods often lack antioxidants, like vitamins C and E, which are vital for fighting oxidative damage (240). Some food additives in processed foods may worsen oxidative stress. These include preservatives and colourants that are pro-oxidants (241). Lastly, processed foods lack dietary fibre and nutrients. This can harm gut health, causing inflammation and oxidative stress (242).

Dr. Robert Lustig, a doctor and researcher, has long fought against processed foods. He perfectly sums up their effects. He explains that, though these foods may contain energy, they prevent our mitochondria from working properly. This causes metabolic dysfunction. As a result, you can't *use* all of the energy they contain (243). Yet your body needs to store the energy somewhere, so it creates fat cells. According to this theory, this is a major reason why processed foods have led to increased rates of overweight and obesity. For this reason, Lustig sees them as *toxins*, not foods. They cause oxidative stress, damage mitochondria, and impair energy production. As outlined before, mitochondrial function is key in autoimmune disease. Metabolic dysfunction contributes to inflammatory gene expression. It is thought to downregulate anti-inflammatory genes and upregulate pro-inflammatory ones.

Bottom line: **stay away from processed foods**.

Prepare as much food yourself as possible. There will be times when you need a quick solution, and or your options are limited. In those instances, do whatever you need to do. But, for most of the time, your meals must be nutritious. They should come from real, minimally processed foods.

You Can't Function Without Protein

When it comes to what we should most definitely have in the diet, my number one recommendation is protein. Your body is 20% proteins. They are in every cell (244). The word protein means "of primary importance" in Greek (245).

Thriving is impossible without dietary protein. Though you can get by with varying levels of carbs and fats as fuel sources, the amount of protein that you consume is critical.

A low-protein diet can cause oxidative stress for several reasons, as I'll outline below.

1. Nervous system function and mood

As explained before, it's vital to balance the ANS. It means having the right activity level in the PNS and SNS. Protein malnutrition can cause autonomic dysfunction. It leads to an overactive SNS and an underactive PNS. This is due to various interconnected mechanisms.

For example, proteins are composed of linked amino acids. They're essential for synthesising neurotransmitters. Tyrosine and tryptophan, both amino acids, are precursors for dopamine and serotonin, respectively. Dopamine is further converted to norepinephrine, which plays a key role in regulating the SNS. A lack of tyrosine can lower dopamine, disrupting norepinephrine levels and over-activating the SNS in a compensatory response.

Similarly, serotonin, which influences mood and the ANS, is produced from tryptophan. Low serotonin can reduce parasympathetic activity. This may cause autonomic dysfunction (246; 247). Conditions like depression, anxiety, PTSD, eating disorders, ADHD, and premenstrual dysphoric disorder (PMDD) are linked to issues with serotonin (248; 249; 250; 251).

Something else that may play a role in the stress response is signalling from neurons in the ENS. Some researchers suspect that a lack of animal protein in a meal triggers signals from the ENS and that these signals prompt us to keep foraging for food until we meet our protein needs. However, the research that led to this conclusion is yet to be peer-reviewed and published, so their suspicion is yet to be verified (252). Meanwhile, Australian researchers have found evidence that we evolved as animal protein hunters and scavengers as part of our omnivorous diet (253). We love sugar and fat. However, hunger is never properly satisfied unless you eat enough high-quality protein. The SNS activation in protein malnutrition may keep you motivated to find more, higher-quality food (i.e. protein), which can be a factor leading to obesity

2.   Cognitive function

Proteins are vital for cognitive function. They help with neuroplasticity. This refers to the brain's ability to adapt and reorganise itself in response to experiences and environmental changes (254). Neuroplasticity is the creation of new neural connections and pathways. They are vital for learning, memory, and brain function.

Protein supports these processes. It provides amino acids needed for neurotransmitter synthesis. It also maintains the structural integrity of neurons. Research shows that protein undernutrition alters brain protein levels, harming motor skills and slowing cognition (255).

If you have "brain fog," it may be due to low protein. Brain fog means you're not functioning at your best. It may be a sign that your brain's neuroplasticity is compromised, and this impairment can limit the brain's ability to adapt to stress. It may also affect the balance of the ANS (256).

Various neurological conditions have been linked to dysregulated neuroplasticity. This includes autoimmune diseases. Your brain's ability to control immune responses and maintain homeostasis may be impaired (257). Also, your reduced ability to learn and adapt may entrench unhealthy behaviours. These include overreactions to non-threatening situations, which can lead to further oxidative stress.

3. Energy production

Protein malnutrition reduces amino acid levels. This affects energy metabolism and limits energy production from non-carb macronutrients as well as other processes. This deficiency can cause hypoglycaemia or low blood sugar, which triggers a stress response. Hypoglycaemia activates the SNS as the body tries to mobilise glucose, which then increases the release of hormones like adrenaline and cortisol. Their chronic release further stimulate the SNS and inhibit the PNS (246).

4. Immune system function

Not getting enough protein can weaken the immune system. This makes you more likely to get infections and experience chronic inflammation. As you know, inflammation can upset the nervous system's balance. This imbalance can harm the body's ability to fight disease and restore homeostasis (246).

5. Antioxidant synthesis

Protein deficiency can lead to a diminished capacity to synthesise antioxidants. Many people don't realise that your body produces many of the antioxidants it uses in its antioxidant defence system. While antioxidants like Vitamin C, Vitamin E, and grape polyphenols can help reduce ROS and prevent oxidative stress, your body's self-produced antioxidants are even more important (258; 259; 260).

Some key antioxidants made in the body are glutathione, catalase, and superoxide dismutase. They are made from amino acids found in protein-rich foods (261; 262; 263). A low-protein diet weakens your antioxidant system, which then causes oxidative stress and increases the likelihood of an immune response.

6. Heart health and blood pressure

Protein is vital for heart health and stable blood pressure. A key reason is it keeps your blood vessel cells (endothelial cells) healthy. A lack of protein can cause these cells to malfunction. This reduces their ability to produce nitric oxide. Nitric oxide is important as it helps widen blood vessels, allowing better blood flow.

A protein deficiency can lower nitric oxide (not to be confused with nitrous oxide or laughing gas, which is an RS) levels. This may narrow your blood vessels and reduce blood flow. This can then strain your heart and raise your blood pressure over time (246). This impairment can raise vascular resistance, prompting the SNS to become more active in maintaining blood pressure. Protein malnutrition also harms heart muscle function. It reduces heart rate variability (HRV), a sign of autonomic nervous system function. Low HRV often indicates an overactive SNS and underactive PNS (256).

How Much Protein Do You Deed?

How much protein do you need? There are differing opinions on this. The widely accepted minimum amount is 0.8g/kg of lean body mass each day (264). It's important to note this is a minimum, not an optimal amount. The research behind this recommendation was based on young, healthy adult males as subjects (265). For all kinds of reasons, young, healthy men use protein more efficiently than people with mitochondrial dysfunction, women, and those older than 25 (266; 267; 268).

The amount you need to thrive depends on factors like your age, activity level, sex, health, and genes. For instance, men have more lean body mass. They are often assumed to need more protein than women of the same weight and activity level. However, because women have lower testosterone levels than men, they may be less efficient at utilising protein. Thus, women may need more protein per unit of lean body mass (269).

Also, older adults tend to develop sarcopenia. This is due to declines in testosterone and human growth hormone with age. So, protein needs to increase as we age (270).

Those with serious illnesses, like autoimmune diseases, may need more protein. They use it less efficiently and have a higher protein turnover due to inflammation (271). And the more you exercise, especially with strenuous activities like weightlifting or manual labour, the more protein you need (272). Additionally, women and older people may need to eat protein both before and after exercise (within a window of 30-60 minutes on either side of exercise) to preserve lean muscle mass, especially under conditions of strenuous exercise. This also helps keep your nervous system balanced; otherwise, there's a risk that the SNS may become more dominant (273; 274). For younger and middle-aged males, there's far less need to be so stringent with protein consumption on either side of exercise.

Genetic variations can also influence protein metabolism and individual requirements. For instance, variations in genes like ACTN3 and MTHFR can affect how well the body uses dietary protein. They are involved in muscle protein synthesis and amino acid metabolism, respectively. I have a couple of genetic mutations that may affect my ability to build muscle while also increasing muscle fatigue and soreness from exercise (275; 276). Adequate protein can help manage their effects. I notice the difference when there's not enough protein in my diet, especially when I'm active.

The current research shows that healthy adults should eat 1.2 to 2.2 grams of protein per kilogram of lean body weight per day (277). For those in the US, that's around 0.5-1g per pound of lean body weight. Lean bodyweight is your ideal healthy bodyweight. For instance, let's pretend that right now I was carrying some excess unhealthy body weight, which meant that I weighed 68kg. My ideal lean body weight is around 57kg (~125 pounds). So, when I calculate my protein needs based on lean body weight, I'll use 57kg as my benchmark, not 68. That means I need to eat in the range of 68.4-125.4 grams of protein per day.

Animal proteins are the most complete and bioavailable. Our bodies are adapted to digest and use them. Those on a mostly plant-based diet need about 30% more protein because plant proteins have much lower digestible bioavailability. That said, fermentation of plant proteins can improve their absorption and use, you can negate the need to eat more protein by choosing fermented plant protein sources (278; 279).

The 1.2 to 2.2 gm range described above offers enough protein for key body functions. It avoids excess that could strain healthy kidneys. However, evidence suggests that over 3 grams per kilogram of body weight per day could help weight-trained people maximise fat loss (280). Very few studies have tested high protein intake due to concerns about kidney health, yet I suspect that, in the future, the recommended limits may rise again, though it comes with the caveat that you drink plenty of water.

It's Not Just Quantity, it's Quality

Also, it's not just about how much protein you get. A wider range of protein types is better. Your body needs over twenty amino acids to make proteins. They are vital for good health. Your body cannot synthesise nine of these, which are considered essential amino acids: histidine, isoleucine, leucine, lysine, methionine, phenylalanine, threonine, tryptophan, and valine. You can *only* get them from food.

The best sources of complete protein are eggs, fish, and animal meats. They contain all nine essential amino acids in sufficient amounts (281). Quinoa, soy, buckwheat, hemp seeds, and chia seeds are complete, plant-based proteins (282; 283; 284; 285; 286). Some unpublished research also suggests that gut bacteria can synthesise some proteins if you eat enough fibre. Herbivorous animals can do this, but whether or not humans can do so at useful levels is yet to be determined (252).

Foods not listed above have various amino acids, but not all of them, meaning they're not complete. To get all the essential amino acids, you need to eat a mix of protein sources. Different protein types are needed to make glutathione. This is the body's main antioxidant, which I touched on briefly before. Because it's so vital to your redox status, I think it's worth discussing it in more detail. It's crucial to grasp why protein plays such a vital role in our diet.

Glutathione is made from three amino acids: cysteine, glutamate, and glycine (287). Low glutathione levels are linked to autoimmune disease progression (288). I've put these three amino acids and the best sources of them into the table below. Your need for each varies. It depends on your oxidative stress and other factors. So, I can't give you a firm guideline. Instead, try to include, at least once a day, one source of each amino acid. You could also try to add all of them to every meal, but please don't do this at the expense of foods that contain the nine essential amino acids.

Amino Acid	Best sources
Cysteine	Whey protein, poultry, beef, eggs, legumes.
Glutamate	Fermented foods (aged cheeses, soy sauce, vegetables, naturally leavened breads), slow cooked meats, eggs, mushrooms, broccoli, peas. Anything with an umami flavour contains glutamate.
Glycine	Bone broth/bovine collagen, marine collagen, red meat (especially cuts that need to be slow cooked, with lots of interconnective tissue), chicken, turkey, pork, and legumes.

Glutathione is present in meat, especially grass-fed herbivores, and in some vegetables and grains, though it's very sensitive to heat. These are all foods that are usually eaten cooked (289). This makes focusing on eating plenty of the foods listed above, which contain the three amino acids glutathione is made from, a better strategy than trying to eat foods rich in glutathione. This way, your body can manufacture its' own glutathione in the liver, whereas if you focus on foods rich in pre-made glutathione, it probably won't survive however you prepare it.

The Devil is in the Detail When it Comes to Fats

When it comes to fats, there's lots of confusion about what we should and shouldn't eat. Here's a brief overview of what the current research shows.

1. Saturated Fats

Saturated fats have been demonised for years. This is due to decades of questionable research led by Dr. Ancel Keys. He was the US's most influential nutrition 'expert' of the 20th Century. I won't delve too deeply into this. Others have done a great job of debunking the myths about saturated fats. But here it is in a nutshell.

Ancel and his colleague's research in the 1960s, 1970s, and 1980s was funded by the sugar and vegetable oil industries. The data was not only flawed and selective, it was also politically and economically motivated. Following WW11,

Keys and his colleagues blamed the rise in heart disease, now the top cause of death worldwide (290), on saturated animal fats in the diet. Much of their work is now discredited, yet it still forms the basis for many official dietary recommendations.

Unfortunately, many in the medical field accepted Keys' 'findings.' This led to a push for low-fat, low-animal-protein diets. You can see this in the US and Australian food pyramids. The proportion of carbohydrates (especially sugar) crept up. When I was little, I remember seeing boxed cereals and even doughnuts at the bottom of the pyramid.

Meanwhile, the so-called "healthy" fats in the standard American diet (SAD) were mostly hydrogenated oils. These oils, such as corn and soybean oil, go through a stabilisation process that hydrogenates them (291). What this process does is add hydrogen unsaturated fats in oil, converting them into saturated fats, which increases their solidity and shelf life. Partially hydrogenated oils are now banned in the US and other countries due to their health risks. However, fully hydrogenated oils are still allowed in manufacturing (292).

Recent research suggests that saturated fats, a dietary staple for millennia, aren't the villains Keys and his colleagues claimed them to be. They don't contribute significantly to raised low-density lipoprotein cholesterol (LDL-C, the form of cholesterol linked to issues with heart health) levels because your liver will produce less when you're getting more from dietary sources (293). In addition, those people in whom this mechanism doesn't work very well – known as hyper responders –tend to have higher levels of high-density lipoprotein cholesterol (HDL-C, the form of cholesterol that protects your heart), but not so much that it ends up creating other risks (294). If you do have high LDL-C without high enough HDL-C to be protective, experience working with clients has taught me that it's generally due to nutrient deficiencies and/or oxidative stress. I'm not going to go into the complicated science behind this, but what I tend to find is that once nutrient deficiencies are corrected and oxidative stress is reduced, LDL-C will lower naturally. I rarely suggest that a client avoid saturated fats as it has little impact on their serum cholesterol and limit their diet.

Saturated fats can be incredibly good for us. There are a couple of reasons why.

Firstly, they're a superb energy source.

As you now understand, mitochondria are the energy factories inside your cells. They produce ATP, which is the energy currency your cells use to function.

However, this process of generating ATP can produce some RS. You know they can harm cells if they build up. ATP production is vital for cellular energy, and managing RS is also key to cell health (Nelson & Cox, 2008). It's a Goldilocks situation – you want to be able to get enough energy without creating more RS than your antioxidants can handle.

Well, guess what?

Fats produce much more ATP than carbohydrates.

One glucose molecule can produce about 30-32 ATP. This is through glycolysis and the citric acid cycle. In comparison, one molecule of palmitic acid (a common fat in meat) can produce around 106 ATP. Fatty acids generate more acetyl-CoA than glucose. So, they make more ATP. In more familiar terms, each gram of fat gives about nine calories. Each gram of carbohydrate gives about four calories (295). Fats provide more energy per gram, making them a better fuel source for long-term needs.

But here's the real kicker: fat metabolism is much better for our bodies than carbs because there are fewer unpleasant side products of metabolism. It's like burning black coal versus brown coal. Brown coal produces more pollutants, namely greenhouse gas emissions. Black coal produces greenhouse gases, too, but at a much lower rate per unit of energy produced (296). Carbohydrates, like brown coal, are the bigger polluters. They produce more RS in proportion to the amount of energy produced (297; 117).

This means that you get a far better return on investment when you burn fat for fuel rather than carbohydrates.

The best energy sources are the long-chain fatty acids in animal fats. You get more bang for your buck with them. Mitochondria are adapted to better handle long-chain fatty acids. They have enzymes and transporters that help these fatty acids enter the mitochondrial matrix, where they can start the process of being broken down.

That said, mitochondria produce more RS when metabolising long-chain fatty acids than when using short-chain fatty acids, which we get from plants. So, there are pluses and minuses for both plant and animal fats. But the bottom line is that, yes, saturated fats are an excellent fuel source.

One last thing about saturated fats. At rest and during low to moderate exercise, like steady walking or light jogging, your muscles prefer fats as a fuel source (298). This is because fat metabolism so effectively provides long-lasting energy. As discussed, fat metabolism yields more ATP per molecule compared to glucose or glycogen. Glucose and glycogen can still be used for fuel, but your body prefers to spare them.

Why? Because when you're at rest, and you have plenty of oxygen available, you use a cleaner and more efficient fuel source. Carbohydrates are more readily depleted during high-intensity activities when oxygen is scarce and fats can't be oxidised. So, if you do fast running, heavy weight lifting, cycling, or some other form of intense exercise, then your body will use carbohydrates. But the rest of the time, it prefers to fuel itself off fats (299).

2.   Long-chain fatty acids

Long-chain fatty acids are Omega-3 fats found in fish, grass-fed animals, and some plant sources. They're not saturated, so they lack the same health warnings as fats from land animals. Many people are probably deficient in them.

In the context of autoimmune diseases, they're important because they have an anti-inflammatory effect. The problem is that most of us simply don't get enough of them, and we get far more Omega-6 fatty acids than we need (300). These two types of fatty acids have a seesaw relationship because they both act on the immune system but with opposite effects. While Omega-3 is anti-inflammatory, Omega-6 is pro-inflammatory (301).

Without enough Omega-3, it's difficult to tame the immune system. Without enough Omega-6, you can't ramp it up in the first place.

Research suggests that we should be consuming these fats in a ratio of around one. That means for every gram of Omega-6, you should also be consuming one gram of Omega-3 (300). As mentioned, the best sources of Omega-3 are fish and seafood, especially fatty fish. You can also find Omega-3 in meat, especially grass-fed, free-range, or wild meats, and in eggs (free-range and grass-fed are best). Other sources are flaxseeds and walnuts, although they're in a slightly different form to those that come from fish and animals, so your body has to convert them to a more usable form (302; 303). Most of these sources have Omega-6 as well. But the ratio is close to one, so you'll hit the target if you prioritise these foods.

3. Plant fats

Plant oils aren't all bad. The right type in the right context can be healthy. But be selective. They're less stable than saturated fats (with a few exceptions). So, use them sparingly in cooking. Extra virgin olive oil has anti-inflammatory properties (304). I prioritise its use in salads and lightly cooked dishes. I use butter and occasionally coconut oil (which is mostly saturated fats) for anything that needs a longer cooking time or higher heat. If you can access them, then use avocado oil, macadamia oil, tallow, and ghee for cooking. They have higher smoke points and contain fewer inflammatory fats than seed oils, which means they're less likely to generate free radicals and/or contribute to oxidative stress and inflammation (305; 306; 307; 308).

Plant oils are fragile, except for coconut oil. So, store them properly and use them quickly. Store them in a sealed container away from direct sunlight. Don't buy so much that you use the same bottle for a year. If it takes you over 2-3 months to finish a bottle, I suggest buying a smaller quantity next time.

Carbohydrates Are Often Overconsumed but Shouldn't Be Completely Dismissed

Now, I do want to explain that carbohydrates shouldn't be demonised completely. Those of us who need carbohydrates must eat them. I eat a small amount of carbohydrates, and I encourage my clients to eat carbohydrates as well if that's what makes them feel best. But why wouldn't we stop eating them if they can lead to more RS being produced?

Well, for one thing, food should be enjoyed, not simply consumed to meet your macros. You have a happy life to live as well!

Some people, especially women, also do better on a diet that includes some carbs. Many people are anti-carb now because carbs raise serum levels of the hormone insulin. You probably know of it as the substance that people with Type 1 diabetes must inject without exception. Excess consumption can also cause Type 2 diabetes, obesity, and metabolic syndrome.

Insulin's job in the body is to ferry glucose into cells. When glucose enters the bloodstream, it signals the pancreas to secrete insulin. This allows glucose to quickly enter cells. There, it can be used right away or stored for later. But, when the cells have enough energy and glucose, insulin receptors in the membrane are told that the cell doesn't need more insulin. These receptors are conduits that allow glucose to enter the cell. As a result, some of the insulin receptors will be downregulated, and insulin will be turned away.

The cell then becomes what's known as insulin resistant. High blood glucose forces the body to convert and store it as fat (216; 309). This can then lead to RS production. Adipose tissue triggers a low-grade immune response, which raises inflammation (310).

So, while I'm an advocate for carbs, I would say it's important not to eat *too many* carbs. It is protein deficiencies in your diet that leave you feeling hungry, and carbs are not a substitute.

If carbs are in every meal, it will be harder to:

- regulate appetite.

- meet protein needs.

- maintain a steady weight.

- limit oxidative stress.

Insulin's effects also extend beyond glucose regulation. It affects the liver's production of sex hormone-binding globulin (SHBG). This protein binds to sex hormones, like estrogen and testosterone, in the blood. SHBG is a carrier that regulates the hormones' bioavailability by controlling their free (active) and bound forms.

You no doubt know that estrogen is one of the primary female sex hormones. Well, guess what? Changes in SHBG levels drastically alter it. High insulin levels, from a high-carb diet, can lower SHBG, increasing free estrogen levels. Less estrogen is bound, so more is available to act on tissues throughout the body (311; 312).

In women, this can cause menstrual issues and contribute to endometriosis and fibroids. In men, it can lead to reduced testosterone synthesis and a decrease in spermatogenesis (313). Both can reduce fertility and increase the risk of autoimmune disease (314).

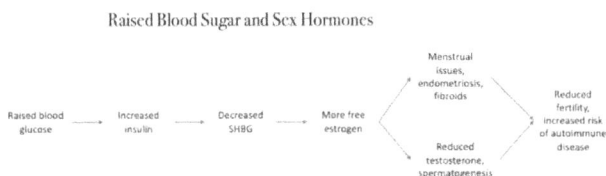

Raised Blood Sugar and Sex Hormones

Raised blood glucose → Increased insulin → Decreased SHBG → More free estrogen → Menstrual issues, endometriosis, fibroids / Reduced testosterone, spermatogenesis → Reduced fertility, increased risk of autoimmune disease

Meanwhile, too little glucose in your blood can also hurt hormonal health. Chronic hypoglycaemia, or low blood sugar, can lower estrogen via several mechanisms. First, it triggers a chain reaction in the body's stress response system. This system is called the hypothalamic-pituitary-adrenal (HPA) axis. It starts with the hypothalamus releasing corticotropin-releasing hormone (CRH). This tells the pituitary gland to release adrenocorticotropic hormone (ACTH). ACTH then signals the adrenal glands to make cortisol.

High cortisol levels can disrupt the hypothalamic-pituitary-gonadal (HPG) axis, which controls reproductive hormones, including estrogen. Cortisol reduces the release of gonadotropin-releasing hormone (GnRH) from the hypothalamus. GnRH is important. It instructs the pituitary gland to release hormones. These include luteinizing hormone (LH) and follicle-stimulating hormone (FSH), both of which are needed for estrogen and testosterone production. As such, chronic hypoglycaemia can disrupt the normal production of testosterone and estrogen (315; 316).

Low Blood Sugar and Sex Hormones

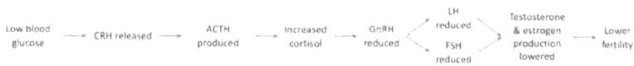

In women, in particular, a lack of energy can worsen this situation by suppressing estrogen, reducing fertility further. In this case, the body's focus shifts from reproduction to survival (317). From an evolutionary view, this is an adaptive response. It helps a woman survive famines so she can reproduce later when food is plentiful, and she and her baby are less likely to starve (318).

As a result, women tend to feel the effects of low blood sugar a little more keenly than men.

One last thing to note on blood glucose. It helps convert thyroxine (T4) into triiodothyronine (T3). T4 is the inactive form of thyroid hormone. T3 is the active and more potent form. If you have Hashimoto's Thyroiditis and/or Graves' Disease (yes, it's possible to have both!), you know how important thyroid hormones are. If you're unfamiliar with the thyroid gland, it produces hormones. They, especially T3, help regulate energy use and ATP production (319). We cannot survive without T3.

T4 conversion to T3 takes place mainly in the liver and kidneys. This involves enzymes called deiodinases. They depend on glucose for energy and as a substrate. Glucose provides the energy for the reactions that convert it. These reactions ensure that T3 levels are sufficient. T3 regulates metabolic processes, such as protein synthesis and lipid metabolism. It also affects mitochondrial function, so it is crucial for energy production and overall health (319). For this reason, I don't recommend a ketogenic diet for most people with hypothyroidism and Hashimoto's, though a low-carb diet that forces their body to prioritise where carbohydrates are used may be useful.

So, as you can see, stable blood glucose levels are vital. They provide energy to cells and optimise thyroid hormones like T3 in tissues. This ensures proper metabolism and good health.

The problem is that women don't burn glucose as well as men. We're much better at burning fat (320; 321). This is likely an adaptive mechanism that increased our chances of survival and reproduction when food was scarcer than today (322).

So, all of this isn't to say that you need to eat loads of carbs or that you need to eat them at every meal. Quite the opposite. It's a balancing situation with blood sugar and insulin. We need a little bit, but not too much.

The best strategy for achieving this is to create a slow, steady release of glucose into your blood. This keeps your blood sugar stable, your cells insulin-sensitive, and hormone production on a nice, even keel. If you eat carbs, do so with or after some protein and fat. This will slow their release into your bloodstream. You'll get a gentle rise in blood sugar, not a sharp spike, which can leave you in a coma an hour later. It will help balance hormones better. And, because of its effects on the nervous system, stable blood sugar lowers inflammation. This means less immune activity (323; 324).

A keto or carnivore diet will still raise your blood glucose and insulin levels when you eat protein. However, blood sugar will rise much less on a low-carb diet (325). Your ability to maintain hormonal health depends on your genetics, insulin sensitivity, and diet. I love vegetables and a wider array of foods too much to do either diet long-term. Though I love to eat meat, I don't personally follow a keto or carnivore diet. And when I tried keto in the past, my body wasn't happy. I suspect this is because of its effects on thyroid hormones, as well as the extra load that fats can place on the liver. I do much better on a low to moderate protein diet with plenty of fruit and vegetables, plus some additional complex carbs because I'm so active.

But know that it is possible. Many people follow keto or carnivore diets with great success. Why are these diets beneficial for so many people? We still need good long-term data on this, but I would guess that it's because there's so much of an emphasis on meats in both diets, and meat provides protein but it's also nutrient-dense. We're about to discuss micronutrients, so what I'm saying here will make more sense once we've had that discussion. But the bottom line is that I believe the more micronutrient-dense your diet is, the less likely you are to run into health issues.

At the same time, it's important to acknowledge that many eat carb-rich diets with great success. The right diet for you depends a lot on genetic factors, as well as age, nutritional status, and activity levels.

A quick note for those wanting to try a carnivore diet. My big tip for success on the carnivore diet is to eat organ meats (and especially liver), not just muscle meat. They should be from grass-fed animals. Beef and other types of red meat are particularly important. If you have certain methylation polymorphisms, red meat can help prevent deficiencies in folate, B12 and other B vitamins needed for methylation pathways (326; 327). These pathways are also crucial for antioxidant pathways and detoxification systems (which you're going to learn all about in the final section of this book).

Tiny But Mighty Micronutrients

Micronutrients are essential nutrients. Your body needs them in small amounts. They are critical for growth, development, and health. Unlike macronutrients, which provide energy (carbs, proteins, and fats), micronutrients do not. They are vital for many body functions and processes.

There are two main categories of micronutrients: vitamins and minerals.

Vitamins are organic compounds. They are coenzymes or precursors in metabolic pathways. These pathways are vital for metabolism, growth, and immunity. Vitamins are of two types. Fat-soluble vitamins A, D, E, and K are stored in the body's fatty tissues and liver. Water-soluble vitamins, like vitamin C and B-complex vitamins (B1, B2, B3, B6, B12, folate, and biotin), dissolve in water. They are not stored in large amounts in the body.

Minerals are inorganic elements. They are vital for many body functions. These include bone formation, nerve function, and enzyme activity. The body requires large amounts of major minerals, such as calcium and magnesium. The body requires trace minerals, such as iron and zinc, in smaller quantities. Both are essential (328; 329).

A consistent issue I see with clients – both those with an autoimmune condition and those who come to me with other issues – is that they have micronutrient deficiencies and concurrent heavy metal toxicity. I've even experienced this myself; I was deficient in zinc, copper, and D3 and suspected long-term folate deficiency, which had only recently been corrected. After reviewing the links between these deficiencies and my symptoms, I decided to check for heavy metal toxicity with a hair mineral analysis. Lo and behold, I had extremely high levels of barium, cobalt, and strontium, and moderately high levels of a couple of others. I don't think it's because I've been exposed to these in excess. I think it's because I've had micronutrient deficiencies that have led to their accumulation. How? Because the micronutrients I was deficient in are so important for producing antioxidants and/or maintaining a balance of these heavy metals. In addition, I had high magnesium levels, which I suspect may have been a sign of my body trying to buffer the effects of having these high heavy metals to alleviate stress on my kidneys, but may also have been related to the cellular effects of chronic activation of the inflammatory reflex on calcium and magnesium levels.

Everyone I work with who has a chronic health issue has trace element deficiencies and/or electrolyte imbalances in conjunction with heavy metal toxicity. These aren't all people with autoimmune diseases. But they all have health issues linked to redox balance.

What's more, a 2015 study highlighted a relationship between antibodies and mercury levels (330). The researchers tested 1352 American women for antinuclear antibodies (ANA), as well as testing their urinary, blood, and hair mercury levels.

What did they find? 16% of women tested positive for ANA. Of that 16%, 96% of them had a speckled staining pattern, indicating autoimmune activity. There was a close relationship between mercury levels in blood and hair (but not urine) and ANA positivity. In fact, the higher the mercury level in blood and hair, the higher the ANA levels.

What this study suggests is that there's a close relationship between the body's ability to detox heavy metals and immune dysregulation. The fact that the relationship was consistent in both blood and hair samples but not urine samples shows that this was a long-term issue, the result of chronic and pervasive exposure. It wasn't about what they'd eaten in the last few days but what their body was grappling with consistently. Furthermore, some of these women had subclinical ANA levels, and their mercury levels were within the accepted range. This means that mercury toxicity, even within accepted ranges, may be predictive of autoimmune disease risk.

What's more, some research suggests that the specific type of heavy metal that accumulates may play a determining role in which autoimmune disease you develop and which organs and tissues are targeted by antibodies. For instance, iron accumulation and iron-mediated programmed cell death (known as ferroptosis) in renal tubules in the kidneys may play a role in the development and pathogenesis of systemic lupus erythematosus and lupus nephritis (331). Meanwhile, cadmium accumulation is a likely mediator of autoimmune tissue or organ damage in tissues and organs where it accumulates (332). While cadmium is cited as an example in the study I've referenced here, the authors stress that it's exactly that: an example. It's possible, perhaps even likely, that any heavy metal that accumulates in quantities that disrupt mitochondrial function and promote ROS production in specific tissues and organs may induce or contribute to autoimmunity. Think back to when we discussed mitochondrial function in the first section of the book – mitochondria actively recruit the immune system when they're under oxidative stress. It's yet to be proven, but I suspect that mitochondrial dysfunction that arises from the accumulation of heavy metals can provoke a mitochondria-mediated immune attack. Unfortunately, heavy metals aren't pathogens, so the damage done by the attack only harms you, not the source of mitochondrial dysfunction. Our bodies have never been subject to so much oxidative stress before now, so they don't have the language to communicate about what's really going on, nor the tools to deal with it.

Why do these heavy metals accumulate? Micronutrients like zinc, copper, B vitamins, and selenium are vital for the proper function of detoxification genes, which we discussed way back in the genetics chapter. A lack of any crucial micronutrient *relative to your body's needs* can be enough to set off a chain reaction that impairs detoxification (333). Our demand for these micronutrients changes when we're under additional stress of some sort – when any of the five pillars of Ecological Nutrition changes our redox balance without an accompanying and equivocal change in dietary substrates needed for detoxification.

For example, many people are currently struggling with detox issues with sulphites and sulphate sensitivity. Common symptoms include nausea post-meals and food sensitivities. The former is indicated by sensitivity to processed foods and wine, especially white wine. The latter is indicated by gastrointestinal discomfort or headaches after eating foods like onion, garlic, and eggs. Other symptoms are hives, rashes, irregular bowel movements, and hormone imbalances. It's not by accident that some people have these issues. Getting the correct nutrition for their needs – micronutrients like vitamin C, magnesium, molybdenum, and the amino acids involved in glutathione production – would have prevented them from developing these sensitivities originally.

In addition, nutrient deficiencies can impact mitochondrial function, leading to reduced energy production and increased oxidative stress. For example, while iron excess is problematic, iron deficiency has also been shown to reduce the efficiency of the electron transport chain, a crucial process in mitochondrial energy production (334). The result is damage to mitochondrial DNA, which ultimately has the potential to reduce your ability to get energy from food, plus impair mitochondria's ability to undertake all of the other functions they do in the body. Perhaps because of their effects on mitochondrial function, micronutrient deficiencies have been linked to obesity, while ameliorating them may aid in weight loss (335). If you struggle to lose weight and can't find an obvious reason, then micronutrient deficiencies might be the cause.

The best advice that I can give you right now is to get as many micronutrients into your diet as possible from food (and sunlight!). We are also going to address these issues more directly in the final section of the book, so you'll learn how to reduce or reverse these kinds of sensitivities.

It's worth noting that many micronutrients serve as antioxidants. For example, the majority of my clients have vitamin D3 deficiency. You can produce D3 in the body by absorbing sunlight through your skin. It's also found in food, especially fatty fish and egg yolks (336). D3 inhibits inflammation by blocking inflammatory molecules produced by the immune system, such as those linked to autoimmune disease (337). It also plays an important role in regulating methylation (338). Vitamin D deficiency has been linked to autoimmune diseases like lupus and rheumatoid arthritis. According to Dr Dimitris Tsoukalas, who runs

Hashimoto's-exclusive clinics in Italy and the U.S., *all* his clients are vitamin D deficient (339).

I discovered that I had a D3 deficiency when I did a thorough check of my blood biomarkers when starting my practice. My hair mineral analysis also revealed high levels of calcium, likely partly related to vitamin D deficiency but maybe also from an ongoing failure to resolve the inflammatory reflex. These two biomarkers can often go hand-in-hand because vitamin D facilitates calcium absorption in the gut (340). If calcium absorption is impaired, then the body will pull calcium from bones to try and maintain calcium homeostasis in tissues, sometimes causing an imbalance that goes the other way, especially if K2 intake or its creation in the gut is poor, especially when under chronic stress. Ultimately, this can result in mitochondrial dysfunction.

There is some debate about how much vitamin D we need. Dr. John Campbell suggests we should take 5 000-50 000 IUs/day (341). This is 125-1250mcg/day, much higher than the accepted limits. I suspect that these recommendations will be revised upwards in the coming years (342; 343). That said, be careful. Some people may need these high amounts of D3 because of a genetic predisposition to not being able to absorb or properly utilise D3. Others may find that 1 000-5 000IUs are plenty. Check your D3 levels and your risk of deficiency before starting any supplements. Too much vitamin D can be just as problematic as not enough.

A note on this, though: standard lab ranges are not suitable for determining if your vitamin D levels are sufficient. Most of the lab ranges I've seen say that anywhere from 30-

50nmol/L is adequate. I strongly disagree as all of my clients (and myself) tend to feel much better when their vitamin D is at least 100nmol/L. My observations also show that many other biomarkers, especially serum lipid profiles, tend to improve with vitamin D at or higher than 100nmol/L. In addition, an expert panel agreed that 80nmol/L is the *minimum* concentration for health, though optimal is likely to be higher than that (344).

The best way to get enough micronutrients is to eat a diet rich in a variety of nutrient-dense foods. Animal-based foods are the most nutrient-dense of all. This includes organ meats, muscle meat, eggs, and fish (147; 345; 327). They have complete proteins, trace elements, vitamins, and healthy fats.

Plants contain them, too, but they tend to be less bioavailable to us. Your needs for various micronutrients in plant foods may vary, but of all the various plant foods, I consider dark leafy greens, berries, and legumes to be the most nutritious. They contain antioxidants and vitamins, plus fibre, which is good for microbiome health (346; 347). That said, you can have normal bowel movements without fibre. Some people also experience better gut health with less fibre in their diets because of genetic predispositions to not being able to break down some fibrous compounds (348; 349). A diet with adequate fat and good hydration help if you don't want to or are unable to eat plenty of fibre-rich foods. However, a diverse microbiome predicts healthy aging and lower oxidative stress (350; 351). And microbes do love fibre. So, it's something to keep in mind.

In areas with poor soils, like some parts of Australia, people might need to take vitamin and mineral supplements. This is because local crops don't have enough nutrients due to the depleted soil. Plants grown in such soils absorb fewer nutrients, leading to deficiencies in vitamins (like D, B, and C) and minerals (like selenium, zinc, and iodine) in both the plants and the animals consuming them. As a result, people may not get enough nutrients from food alone, so supplementation helps ensure proper nutrition and prevents health issues (352).

As an anecdotal aside, I see loads of people with zinc deficiency in Australia, which can manifest as things like issues with lipid metabolism, iron deficiency, issues with leaky gut and bowel movements, and hormonal imbalances. Zinc is crucial to so many processes in the body (including management of oxidative stress), and our soils here are so deficient that it can become a major problem. While many of them are anaemic, it's not necessarily because they're not getting enough iron; it's because they can't store and use it without zinc. Along with vitamin D3 and B vitamin deficiencies in general, particularly in the area where I live, which is very cold and often overcast, this has been the most consistent deficiency I've seen in my Australian clients.

Also, dietary preferences, food processing, and seasonal availability can affect nutrient intake. So, supplementation is a practical way to meet nutritional needs – just make sure it doesn't become a stand-in for a micronutrient-rich diet (353).

The best way to know if you need to supplement is to get relevant testing done. You might suspect what you're deficient in. But it's hard to know without checking. Some micronutrients can be harmful in high doses. So, it's safest to check first.

It's important, though, to note your testing might not show any micronutrient deficiencies. The reason why is that lab ranges are based on statistical significance for *disease*, not optimal health. Think back to the vitamin D example I mentioned earlier. Even though research shows the requirement for health is higher than that stated by the lab, the lab ranges don't reflect this.

The reason why lab ranges can fail to pick up on nutrient deficiencies or issues is because of how they're established. You might be getting less than you need of something. But, it's not so much less that you end up with a diagnosable condition that research has linked to it.

For example, many of my clients have low alkaline phosphatase, which is a biomarker of liver function. I also use it as a functional biomarker for zinc status. Their zinc deficiency isn't so bad that their alkaline phosphatase falls outside of lab ranges, but it's lower than optimal. It falls outside *my* range. So, it won't be highlighted as deficient in your regular lab work. I'll mention this again later because it's so important, but you must work with someone who can look at your lab tests and compare them against optimal levels.

I also have a small e-book that teaches you how to read your general blood tests and decipher what you might need some more of if you'd rather go it alone – you can find it by searching me on Amazon or looking at the books tab on my website. It's called "How to Interpret Your Blood Test Results".

Unfortunately, a wholly plant-based diet will require you to supplement to meet your micronutrient needs. Some micronutrients are usually higher in animal-based foods. For example, B12 is only found in animal products. If you don't eat meat or animal products, then you will need to supplement it (354). Vitamin D is another critical nutrient to check on and supplement if needed, especially if sunlight is limited. It's mainly found in animal products, and animal fats can help with its synthesis in the body (355).

Omega-3 fatty acids EPA and DHA are vital for heart and brain health, as well as proper immune system regulation. They are mainly in fish and seafood. Plant sources, like flaxseeds and chia seeds, provide ALA. The body can convert ALA to EPA and DHA, though it's not a very efficient process. Only around 10% of ALA is converted to EPA and 2-5% of that to DHA (356; 357).

Iron from plants (non-heme iron) needs careful planning. It requires vitamin C-rich foods to boost absorption (358). Also, a plant-based diet can make it hard to get enough calcium, zinc, and iodine. Depending on individual needs, supplements may again be needed (359). Again, it's important to test and track your levels. This is to avoid getting too low or too high from inappropriate supplements.

Boost Your Energy Levels with Creatine

Creatine is a beneficial supplement for many people with autoimmune diseases. It's a relatively safe compound made naturally in the liver, kidneys, and pancreas from amino acids and is primarily stored in muscle cells. It plays a key role in energy production, especially for short bursts of activity like weightlifting or sprinting, by boosting ATP levels, the primary energy source for cells. Research supports its effectiveness in improving muscle strength, power, and exercise performance, particularly when combined with resistance training. Creatine also aids muscle recovery and promotes muscle growth (360; 361; 362).

You may wonder why I recommend something that sounds best for gym jocks looking to get huge. There are a couple of reasons. The main one is energy production. Autoimmune conditions cause inflammation, which is energetically costly. As I'm sure you've experienced, this weakens muscles and causes fatigue. Creatine supplementation supports muscle function and improves energy levels. In doing so, it can alleviate symptoms associated with autoimmune disease, including what's colloquially known as "brain fog" (363; 364). New research suggests creatine may also reduce inflammation by acting as an antioxidant (365).

Before taking creatine, I recommend checking with your doctor. Because it's excreted through the kidneys, it can add a little extra stress on them. If you have severe kidney issues, it may not be safe for you.

If you do take it, hydrate properly. It works by shuttling water into cells, which reduces circulating water in the body. You then become more prone to dehydration, which is why it can strain the kidneys.

The correct dose of creatine varies according to what you're hoping to achieve. To gain muscle and boost energy, 5g/day should suffice. But I recommend starting with 1g/day. Then, increase to 5g over a few weeks to let your body adjust. Keep track of how you're feeling and lower the dose if you notice any negative side effects. For those wanting to enjoy creatine's brain benefits, a higher dose of 10g/day may be better. This is especially true if you have poor methylation. Again, be cautious. Work your way up to avoid an upset stomach and back it off if need be.

Fabulous Fibre

I've talked a bit about gut health. Here, I want to focus on the link between the microbiome and fibre consumption. All the food categories we've discussed can affect your microbiome. But fibre deserves some recognition on its own.

I first realised the importance of fibre to microbes, not through study or my health, but by fermenting honey-based alcohols called ambrosia. I saw the ferments were much slower than wine ferments. But when I added botanicals or infusing agents, they sped up a lot. After some research, I found that the added fibre was likely the main reason. The yeast doing the fermentation was a lot happier when it was in there.

Within your gut, you also have what's known as the gut microbiome. This is a collection of billions of single-celled organisms, yeast and bacteria. They help you digest food. They mostly produce the gut's neurotransmitters and hormones. They affect your emotions and send signals to the brain (366). The healthier and happier they are, the better off they'll be, both mentally and physically (367).

Your gut microbiome also helps regulate your immune system (368). We've already discussed, way back in the chapter on the immune system, that the majority of the innate immune system is housed in the gut. If microbes in your gut think something is wrong, then they're much more likely to kick up a fuss and get the immune system involved.

This means that dysbiosis, or microbial imbalance, can play a causal role in autoimmune diseases. It does this by increasing intestinal permeability, leading to chronic inflammation (368; 369). We already discussed this with stress and gluten. But it's not *just* about keeping the wrong things out. A well-functioning gut needs enough fibre.

Dietary fibre in fruits, vegetables, legumes, and whole grains, feeds good gut bacteria. These bacteria ferment dietary fibre. They produce short-chain fatty acids (SCFAs), including butyrate, propionate, and acetate (370).

SCFAs are crucial for gut health. They help maintain your gut barrier, reducing leaky gut (371). A healthy gut barrier stops antigens and pathogens from entering the bloodstream and triggering autoimmune responses. Also, SCFAs can reduce inflammation and modulate immune responses, which can help with autoimmune diseases (372).

Fibre-rich diets support gut bacteria that boost Tregs, immune cells that prevent autoimmunity by promoting self-tolerance (373; 374). A high-fibre diet can also create a diverse microbiome, improving immune regulation and reducing the risk of autoimmune diseases.

How much you should have depends on your size. The current recommendation is from 25-38 g per day (375) The smaller you are, the lower the recommendation is. That said, there is evidence that a higher intake of up to 50g per day is beneficial (376). This may be especially important as you get older.

Unless you're on a carnivore diet or don't do well with plant foods, eat more fibre. Or, unless you eat chia seeds by the cupful, you'll struggle to get enough fibre. It's unlikely you'll get too much.

Here are some of the most fibre-rich foods to include in your diet, including their fibre content (377; 378).

- Chia seeds: 34.4g/100g
- Flaxseeds: 27.3g/100g
- Split peas: 25g/100g
- Black beans: 15.2g/100g
- Chickpeas: 12.5g/100g
- Nigella seeds: 10.5g/100g (these are also the source of "black seed oil", which has strong antioxidant properties)
- Artichokes: 8.6g/100g
- Lentils: 7.9g/100g

I recommend starting slow by adding more fibre to your diet. Your microbiome will need a little bit of time to reproduce and readjust, so add an extra 3-5g/day in weekly increments until you hit your target. For instance, if you currently eat around 20g/of fibre per day, spend a week eating 23-25g per day. The next week, aim for 28-30g per day. And so on.

One of the Best Ways to Nourish Yourself Is... Not Eat

One last thing I want to touch on here is the timing of eating. Fasting is a hot topic in nutrition and weight loss. It's gained attention for several reasons. Let's quickly go over what happens when you fast. This will help you decide how you want to approach it.

We have discussed how metabolism causes the production of ROS. If you keep metabolising without letting your mitochondria rest, it can create more oxidative stress. This is due to errors in metabolism. With that in mind, let's consider a shorter fast, like overnight. What might it do for us?

Overnight fasting – between dinner and breakfast – is a time for your body to rest from breaking down food for energy. Your mitochondria can use stored food as fuel if needed. But their energy demands are usually lower at night. You should be asleep or at least in a state of deep rest, which will be accompanied by a slowdown in energy production that allows the mitochondria to focus on other tasks. These include repairing mitochondrial DNA and clearing debris, including ROS, from the cell (379; 380). It's like doing the dishes each day. Then, you can cook without dodging a cluttered kitchen or using dirty pots and pans. This makes cooking more seamless.

During long fasts, like 24–48 hours, mitochondria will degrade faulty ones and recycle their parts for use in other mitochondria. This process is called mitophagy (381). This allows mitochondria's life and usefulness to the cell to extend. Think of the DNA repairs like getting regular oil changes in your car. The better you care for the engine, the better the car will run. It will last longer and burn fuel more cleanly.

And finally, fasting can catalyse mitochondrial biogenesis. This is how cells make new mitochondria. There are a couple of mechanisms by which fasting promotes mitochondrial biogenesis. Fasting activates AMP-activated protein kinase (AMPK), a cellular energy sensor. When it senses low energy in the cell, AMPK activates. It stimulates mitochondrial biogenesis by increasing the expression of genes involved in the process. This creates more mitochondria to boost energy production (382).

Fasting also boosts the production of Nicotinamide adenine dinucleotide (NAD+), a molecule that signals the body's energy status. When energy is low, higher NAD+ levels activate genes that produce enzymes called sirtuins, like SIRT1. These enzymes are vital for many cell functions, including making new mitochondria. This process helps cells produce energy more efficiently during fasting (383).

The other wonderful thing about sirtuin genes is their role in reducing inflammation (384). They do this in part through a synergy with erythroid 2–related factor 2 (Nrf2). Nrf2 is a molecule that regulates antioxidant and detoxification genes. It boosts your antioxidant defence system and reduces oxidative stress. When you fast, SIRT1 stabilises and boosts Nrf2. This raises the activity of the detox and antioxidant genes that Nrf2 targets (385). Exercise and low oxidative stress from antioxidants in foods like turmeric also trigger the production of sirtuin enzymes (386; 387). You can also take nicotinamide mononucleotide (NMN), a precursor to NAD+, to boost sirtuin production. Yi and colleagues (2023) have proven NMN to be highly effective as a supplement at dose rates up to 900mg.

Now, all this isn't to say that you should be fasting for extended periods each day or doing a two-day fast every month. What type of fasting each of us should practice depends on a lot of different factors.

Age is a big one. Children have higher rates of mitophagy and mitochondrial biogenesis than adults. A quick recap on these terms: mitophagy is the process of breaking down mitochondria and reusing parts for repairs in other mitochondria, while mitochondrial biogenesis is the process of making new mitochondria.

Children's higher rates of mitophagy and mitochondrial biogenesis are due to several factors. One is the rapid growth and development that children undergo. During growth, your cells need more energy. So, they must remove damaged parts and produce new ones. These processes can decline with age. Causes include cellular damage, lifestyle factors, and metabolic changes (388). Fasting in its various forms can thus become more important as we age.

That said, fasting can be stressful. It may increase sympathetic tone in the ANS, especially if done for too long or too often. Shorter-duration fasts, known as time-restricted feeding (TRF), are generally recommended for those with less body fat (389). In addition, women's hormone balance, influenced by blood sugar, suffers with extended daily fasting. 12-14 hours is generally best for women. Biological males, on the other hand, may get benefits from fasting for up to 16 hours or even longer (390). So, the best way to gain fasting's benefits is to practice TRF regularly, based on what's most appropriate to your biological sex.

Longer fasts, over 24 hours, can be beneficial but should be done only *occasionally* (391). How often is very dependent on you as a person. Before starting an extended fast, check with your functional or holistic healthcare provider. They can review your blood tests to see if it's safe and likely to help.

One last note on fasting. Some truly astounding research on fasting is emerging. It shows that the benefits of fasting may also be achieved through fasting-mimicking diets, like the keto diet. For example, a 2017 study tested a four-day fasting-mimicking diet in mice. They had late-stage Type 1 and Type 2 diabetes from prior treatment, meaning their pancreas had suffered damage from auto-antibody attacks and wasn't functioning well. They were fed a low-protein, nutrient-dense diet that met 50% of their energy needs on day one, then 10% on days two to four. Ten days of normal eating followed. Then, they had to start another round of the fasting-mimicking diet.

The mice had all the usual symptoms of late-stage Type 1 and Type 2 diabetes when the fasting intervention began. They had impaired insulin production and damaged beta cells.

After several rounds of fasting, the mice regenerated their beta cells and fully recovered. The researchers found that the fasting-mimicking diet reactivated specific genes, usually only upregulated during a critical period early in life when the pancreas develops.

The same study found that pancreatic cells from Type 1 diabetes human donors could regenerate beta cells. This was after exposure to a solution with compounds produced by the mice during the fasting-mimicking diet. It upregulated the gene for pancreatic beta cell development (392).

Keep an eye out for updates on fasting. Its role in cell signalling may help those with autoimmune diseases.

Activity

The number one question that I get asked about autoimmune diseases is what someone should eat. I always tell people that this is personal, but there are some general rules.

They can be hard to remember, though. And sometimes, it's hard to spot where you're going wrong. This activity is going to help you synthesise the information you've just learned about diet into an actionable plan for you.

1. *Evaluate Your Nutritional Status*

This self-assessment will help you evaluate your nutritional intake in terms of protein, fat, fibre, micronutrients, and time-restricted feeding habits. Use this as a tool to reflect on your dietary patterns and identify areas for improvement.

Please also note that the following information is general and not intended as medical advice.

Step 1: Protein Intake

1. How many servings of protein do you consume per day?
   - 1-2 servings
   - 3-4 servings
   - 5 or more servings

2. List your typical sources of protein (e.g., meat, eggs, dairy, legumes, nuts, seeds, etc.):

3. Do you consume a variety of protein sources throughout the week (e.g., animal-based, plant-based, fish, and legumes)?
   - Yes
   - No

4. How often do you consume the following protein-rich foods?
   - Meat (beef, chicken, etc.):
     - Daily
     - Weekly
     - Rarely
   - Fish or seafood:
     - Daily
     - Weekly
     - Rarely
   - Plant-based proteins (lentils, beans, tofu, etc.):
     - Daily
     - Weekly

- Rarely

5. Estimate your daily protein intake:
   Aim for 1.2 to 2.2 grams of protein per kilogram of body weight per day OR 0.5 to 1 gram of protein per pound of body weight.
To calculate, multiply your weight (in kg) by 1.2 and 2.2 to get your range or in pounds, by 0.5 and 1.

   Example calculation:
   For a person weighing 70 kg, the range is 84g to 154g, as calculated below.
   70 kg × 1.2 = 84 g
   70 kg × 2.2 = 154 g
   Your range: _____ g to _____ g per day.

6. Are you confident that your diet includes all essential amino acids?
These are histidine, isoleucine, leucine, lysine, methionine, phenylalanine, threonine, tryptophan, and valine.
Ensure your protein sources include a variety of animal and plant-based options to meet all essential amino acids.

Step 2: Fat Intake

1. What are your main sources of fat?
   Tick all that apply:
   - Saturated fats (butter, cream, fatty cuts of meat)
   - Monounsaturated fats (olive oil, avocados)
   - Polyunsaturated fats (fish, flaxseeds, walnuts)
   - Trans fats (fried foods, processed snacks)

- Omega-6 fats (cottonseed oil, sunflower oil, canola oil, grapeseed oil)

2. How often do you consume foods high in omega-3 (e.g., fish, grass-fed red meat, flaxseeds, walnuts)?
  - Daily
  - Weekly
  - Rarely

3. Are your fat sources well-balanced and varied?
  - Well-balanced (a good mix of different fats with little trans or additional omega-6 oils)
  - Somewhat balanced (mixed, but saturated, monounsaturated, and polyunsaturated fats dominate)
  - Unbalanced (reliant on trans and omega-6 fats)

Step 3: Carbohydrate Intake

Carbohydrates are not required for everyone. It's important to reflect on whether you may be over-reliant on them for energy or comfort.

1. What percentage of your daily calories comes from carbohydrates?
  - Less than 30%
  - 30-50%
  - More than 50%

2. List your main sources of carbohydrates:
  - Whole grains (brown rice, oats, quinoa)
  - Refined grains (white bread, pasta)
  - Fruits and vegetables

- Sugary foods (sweets, pastries, etc.)

3. Do you feel reliant on carbohydrates for energy throughout the day?
  - Yes
  - No

4. Do you notice fatigue or energy crashes when you reduce carbohydrates or after meals high in carbohydrates?
  - Yes
  - No

5. Do you balance carbohydrate intake with sufficient protein and fats?
  - Yes
  - Sometimes
  - No

Step 4: Micronutrient Intake

Evaluate your intake of key vitamins and minerals essential for overall health.

1. How often do you consume foods rich in the following micronutrients?

  - Iron (e.g. red meat):
    - Daily
    - Weekly
    - Rarely
  - Zinc (e.g. oysters, beef, chickpeas):
    - Daily

- Weekly
- Rarely
- Magnesium (e.g. dark leafy greens, nuts, seeds):
- Daily
- Weekly
- Rarely
- Vitamin D (e.g. fatty fish, eggs, sun exposure):
- Daily
- Weekly
- Rarely
- Calcium (e.g. dairy, fortified plant-based milk):
- Daily
- Weekly
- Rarely

2. Do you take any vitamin or mineral supplements?
   If yes, list them here: _____

Step 5: Fibre Intake

Fibre is essential for healthy digestion and maintaining regular bowel movements.

1. How many grams of fibre do you estimate you consume daily?
   Aim for 25-50g of fibre per day.
   - Less than 10g
   - 10-20g
   - 20-30g
   - More than 30g

2. What are your primary sources of fibre?

- Seeds and nuts
- Legumes (lentils, beans)
- Vegetables
- Fruits.

3. Do you experience any digestive issues such as constipation or bloating?
   - Yes
   - No

4. Do you consume high-fibre foods daily (vegetables, fruits, legumes)?
   - Yes
   - Sometimes
   - Rarely

Step 6: Time-Restricted Feeding (Intermittent Fasting)

Consider whether intermittent fasting could be beneficial for you. Time-restricted feeding (TRF) refers to eating only during specific windows of time.

1. Do you follow any time-restricted feeding schedule?
   - Yes
   - No

2. How many hours do you fast per day?
   - Less than 12 hours
   - 12-14 hours
   - More than 14 hours

3. Do you notice any benefits (e.g., improved energy, mood, or weight management) from fasting?
   - Yes
   - No

4. Is fasting for at least 12 hours (for women) or 14 hours (for men) sustainable for you?
   - Yes
   - No

Step 7: General Dietary Patterns

1. How often do you eat processed or convenience foods (e.g., fast food, packaged snacks)?
   - Daily
   - Weekly
   - Rarely

2. Do you consume alcohol?
   - Yes: _____ drinks per week
   - No

Results Interpretation

- Protein: Aim to meet the daily protein target (1.2-2.2 g/kg body weight) with a variety of sources.
- Fats: Ensure a balance of healthy fats, including omega-3s.
- Carbohydrates: If you rely heavily on carbs, consider whether you need to adjust your intake for better energy balance. This is particularly relevant if you're often "hangry" or have fluctuations in energy throughout the day. Consider increasing your protein intake.

- Micronutrients: Ensure you are meeting daily needs for key vitamins and minerals through food or supplements.
- Fibre: Target at least 25g of fibre daily from whole foods, more if feasible, *unless* you have a genetic predisposition to not breaking fibre down well or are trying a carnivore diet.
- Time-Restricted Feeding: Consider adopting intermittent fasting if it fits your lifestyle and brings health benefits.

2. Test for Heavy Metals

You've just read how heavy metals can be predictive of autoimmune disease and are present in close to 100% of people with autoimmune antibodies. This means that it's well worth checking if this is you and if you need to do some kind of heavy metal detox (more on how to do this later). A hair mineral analysis will give you the most accurate results – saliva and urine just don't cut it, as they only offer a short-term perspective. The study cited earlier showed that blood can be a good indicator, but I think that hair is the way to go because it gives a long-term snapshot. In addition, it's likely going to be cheaper to test for a wide range of heavy metals with hair analysis compared to blood.

Chapter Summary

- Many dietary factors contribute to oxidative stress. Personalised nutrition is emphasised over prescribing specific diets, as individual needs vary based on individual biology, context, goals, and stage in the autoimmune journey.
- Monitor how food affects you and adjust your diet accordingly. Conditions like SIBO and mould exposure can impact food tolerance and appetite.

- The gut is influenced by mental and emotional stress through the autonomic nervous system (ANS), specifically the enteric nervous system (ENS), which plays a major role in the regulation of the immune system housed in the gut.
- Stress and immune activation can lead to "leaky gut syndrome". Tight junctions in the gut open, allowing toxins and pathogens to enter the bloodstream.
- Gluten, particularly gliadin from wheat, rye, and barley, can affect gut permeability and is linked to chronic health conditions like nutritional deficiencies, osteoporosis, infertility, cancer, and autoimmune diseases.
- Sourdough bread, especially with long fermentation, can break down gluten, reducing its potential negative impact on gut health. Sourdough from supermarkets and large chains may not offer these benefits due to shorter fermentation times and added yeast.
- Processed foods include any packaged foods with multiple ingredients, especially those with lab-synthesised additives not found in nature and should be avoided.
- Protein is crucial for survival and optimal health, forming 20% of the body and essential for neurotransmitter synthesis and autonomic nervous system balance.
- Inadequate protein intake can cause oxidative stress, autonomic dysfunction, cognitive impairment, weakened immune system, disrupted energy metabolism, and cognitive issues.

- Recommended protein intake is 1.2 to 2.2 grams per kilogram of body weight per day, adjusted for age, sex, activity level, and health status.
- Animal proteins, particularly meat, fish, and eggs, are complete and highly bioavailable, which means they're easily used by your body. Plant-based diets may require 30% more protein to compensate for lower bioavailability.
- Glutathione is made from cysteine, glutamate, and glycine. It's an antioxidant critical for combating oxidative stress and supporting immune function.
- Hydrogenated oils, such as corn and soybean oils, pose health risks.
- Recent research suggests saturated fats can be beneficial and are a good energy source.
- Fat metabolism in mitochondria is more efficient than carbohydrate metabolism, producing more energy and fewer reactive oxygen species (ROS).
- Saturated fats are the body's favoured food source during rest and low-intensity exercise, NOT carbohydrates.
- The ideal ratio of omega-6 to omega-3 fatty acids in a diet is about 1:1 – most people are getting more pro-inflammatory omega-6 than anti-inflammatory omega-3.
- Healthy plant oils like extra virgin olive oil have anti-inflammatory properties but should be used with care when cooking due to lower stability at higher temperatures compared to saturated fats. Macadamia and avocado oil are better options for cooking at high temperatures.

- Carbohydrates can be essential for some people, especially women.
- Insulin helps regulate glucose in the blood, but excessive glucose can lead to insulin resistance and fat storage. Carbohydrate intake should be tailored to optimise blood sugar and insulin sensitivity.
- Chronically low blood sugar (hypoglycaemia) can negatively affect hormone production, including estrogen and testosterone.
- Stable blood sugar is important for converting thyroid hormones and ensuring proper metabolic function.
- Slow, steady glucose release from carbohydrates is preferable for stable blood sugar and hormone levels, which can be achieved through fat and protein consumption alongside carbohydrates.
- Micronutrients are essential nutrients required in small amounts for growth, development, and health and include vitamins and minerals.
- People with poor micronutrient status may be at increased risk of developing heavy metal toxicity, which may be a good predictor (and partial cause) of autoimmune disease.
- The most micronutrient-rich food sources are animal-based foods (e.g., organ meats, muscle meat, eggs, fish), while plant foods, dark leafy greens, berries, and legumes also offer antioxidants and vitamins.
- Regions with poor soil might require supplements due to nutrient deficiencies.
- Plant-based diets may need supplementation for vitamin B12, vitamin D, omega-3s, and iron.

- Dietary fibre is crucial for a healthy gut microbiome as it is a key nutrient for beneficial gut bacteria and immune regulation, the best sources are seeds and legumes.
- Short-chain fatty Acids (SCFAs) produced from fibre fermentation, SCFAs help maintain gut barrier integrity and have anti-inflammatory properties.
- Creatine enhances muscle strength, power, and recovery; it may support energy levels and reduce inflammation in autoimmune diseases.
- Short-term fasting (e.g., overnight) allows mitochondria to rest and repair, similar to cleaning up a kitchen after cooking.
- Longer fasting (24-48 hours) promotes mitophagy, where damaged mitochondria are recycled, extending the life of healthy mitochondria, as well as the production of new mitochondria.
- Fasting is potentially more beneficial as we age.
- Fasting duration should be adjusted based on body fat, gender, and individual health; women may need shorter (12-14 hours) overnight fasts compared to men (16+ hours).
- Extended fasts should be occasional and consulted with a healthcare provider.
- Fasting-mimicking diets have the potential to regenerate pancreatic beta cells in diabetes models, indicating possible benefits for organ and gland growth and repair in autoimmune conditions.

How to Clean Up and Beautify Your Environment

"Man's attitude toward nature is today critically important simply because we have now acquired a fateful power to alter and destroy nature. But man is a part of nature, and his war against nature is inevitably a war against himself..."

Rachel Carson

It's no secret that there are many potential hazards in the environment. Environmental factors are related to many conditions, including cancer and autoimmune disease. Their effect on your immune system depends on the toxin or pathogen involved. This effect also depends on how these environmental hazards interact with your immune system and genes.

They can do so many things that affect autoimmune diseases. This includes suppression of your immune system, binding to endocrine and immune system receptors, and turning on genes that promote inflammation. They can also bind to nucleic acids (DNA) and promote anti-nuclear autoimmunity. They can deplete the antioxidant defence system, promote the breakdown of immune barriers, like skin and mucus, and alter normal antigen-presenting responses (393).

We find chemicals everywhere, from personal care and cleaning products right through to the foods you eat, the air you breathe and even in the rain (394; 395; 396; 397). Many of these substances are endocrine disruptors. They directly induce the production of reactive species (RS) in cells.

For example, BPA is plastic in food packaging and receipts. It directly stimulates ROS generation in various cell types. This includes endothelial cells and hepatocytes, the primary functional cells in the liver. Bad news for detoxing RS. Also, phthalates in personal care products and food packaging can impair antioxidant enzymes. Oxidative stress arises because the cell can't counteract RS buildup.

Some endocrine disruptors can also directly harm mitochondria. This, in turn, increases RS production due to faulty metabolism. This oxidative stress can damage DNA, cause inflammation, and harm cells. It raises the risk of diseases from endocrine disruptor exposure (398; 399; 400). These impacts emphasise the need to limit exposure to endocrine disruptors.

Are Household Items Making Your Condition Worse?

I recommend staying away from synthetic cleaning products and switching to more natural brands for personal care and cleaning (or using hot water and a bit of vinegar!). I use hot water and unscented or naturally scented (with essential oils) detergents to clean the house and kitchen.

I think we have an unfounded obsession in our culture with microbial cleanliness. Remember that microbes can be both detrimental and beneficial for your health. You need bacteria in your gut, dental cavity, and even on your skin for optimal health. Recent research has even found that your brain has its microbiome (401). The same chemicals used to kill microbes in your house could harm your microbiome.

Some researchers also suggest a lack of early exposure to germs and parasites raises allergy risk. It may suppress the immune system's natural development. This is the "hygiene hypothesis." According to Dr. David P. Strachan, a cleaner environment, common in developed countries, may raise autoimmune and allergic diseases. He suggested that, though smaller families and better hygiene in the 20th century led to fewer infections, they caused a rise in hay fever and other allergies (402). Our obsession with cleanliness means that the immune system doesn't get enough stimulation to develop properly.

Something else to be aware of in your home and when you do the shopping is plastic. Plastic is everywhere! In his 2022 book, Matt Simon highlights just how pervasive plastics are (403). Not only are they in every household, car, workplace, and even in the rain, but they have invaded our internal organs and tissues as well. They have been found in human reproductive organs, the brain, and even in the first stool samples of newborn babies.

It's impossible to get away from it completely. Yet by reducing the amount of food that you consume that's been wrapped or packaged in plastic, you can significantly reduce your exposure to it. This includes plastic bottled water, takeaway coffee and hot beverages (the paper cups are plastic lined, and heat increases the volatility of the lining, meaning you can end up drinking it), canned foods, and processed foods in general. And, because our oceans are so heavily polluted with plastics, sea salt is also often contaminated with plastics, meaning that it's no longer truly safe to consume.

If you use or come into contact with a lot of plastic in your day-to-day life, I strongly recommend making as many switches as feasible to reduce your exposure to plastics.

For self-care, use honey as a facial cleanser and tallow as a moisturiser. Or switch to low-tox personal care brands. There are plenty on the market now. Examine the back labels of every product thoroughly. Among the most problematic endocrine disruptors in personal care products are:

- Phthalates are plasticisers and fragrance carriers. Dodson et al. (404). have linked them to reproductive disorders, as they disrupt hormone production.
- Parabens are common preservatives. They mimic estrogen and may disrupt hormones, raising breast cancer risk (405).
- Triclosan is an antibacterial product. It disrupts thyroid function and hormone signalling (406).
- Bisphenol A (BPA) can mimic estrogen and disrupt hormones. Some cosmetics and packaging use it. It's now less common in cosmetics due to regulations, but you will still find it in a lot of packaging (407).
- Some cosmetics may contain heavy metals (lead, mercury, arsenic, and cadmium). They can

accumulate in the body and disrupt the endocrine system, posing serious health risks (408).

Avoid products with these chemicals. Choose natural or organic cosmetics instead.

Chemicals in Food Are Far More Harmful Than We're Told

With food, it's best to buy organic when possible. Better yet, buy from someone you trust not to use synthetics. It's okay if they aren't certified organic. Or grow your own. Farmers spray various synthetic chemicals, such as herbicides and pesticides, on foods. Glyphosate, or Roundup™, isn't the most lethal chemical in food production. But it's worth examining what we know about it because is it the most widely used. It's useful to understand how agricultural chemicals are approved for use and monitored.

In 1974, the market introduced glyphosate as a broad-spectrum weed killer. Since then, it has become the most used chemical in agriculture. Monsanto assured everyone it was safe for humans. I've heard of sales reps from Monsanto telling farmers it was so safe they could drink it!

This is false and misleading. No one in their right mind would drink glyphosate, for good reason.

Glyphosate is water-soluble and is absorbed and transported in organic tissues with ease. It blocks a growth-related enzyme in plants, fungi, and bacteria which acts through the shikimate pathway. This leads to the organism's death. As a non-selective herbicide, it kills any exposed plant or microorganism (409).

Scientists have developed genetically modified (GM) crops that are resistant to glyphosate, leading to an increased use of this herbicide. This allows farmers to protect their crops from weeds more effectively, enabling them to apply herbicides without damaging the crops themselves. As a result, the cultivation process becomes more efficient and sustainable, helping to enhance crop yields and manage weed populations more effectively (410).

The problem is that these crops can absorb glyphosate but not metabolise it. This leaves trace amounts in food. In 2018, traces were found in 43 of 45 US breakfast cereals (411).

Though strict guidelines exist for glyphosate use in agriculture, adherence is not always guaranteed. Farmers sometimes use glyphosate outside its approved periods to maximise yield (412). There are also examples of it being found in organic wine, indicating that it's not being properly used (413).

Health risks are debated. The IARC classified glyphosate as "probably carcinogenic" in 2015, citing links to non-Hodgkin lymphoma. Agrochemical companies have challenged this finding. But animal and community studies support it (414; 415; 416). One of glyphosate's derivatives, aminomethylphosphoric acid (AMPA), has been found in human blood following poisonings (417). Studies also link glyphosate to oxidative stress, DNA damage, increased birth defects, and increased ADHD rates (418; 419; 420; 421).

The reason why it slips through the cracks in research on safety is simple. Glyphosate's formulations, like Roundup, are more potent than glyphosate alone. They contain added surfactants (422). These formulations are up to *100 times* more effective. Company-published research only tests glyphosate in isolation (423). This approach has a purpose.

In 2018, a US court ruled that Monsanto (now Bayer) caused a man's cancer due to glyphosate. It awarded him significant damages (424). Internal documents showed Monsanto ignored warnings and rigged studies to downplay glyphosate's risks (425). They've been aware of the risks for a long time. Despite this, glyphosate remains legal in most countries.

You can't necessarily trust governments and regulatory bodies to protect you from the interests of big business. At this point, it's up to you to protect yourself.

Folic Acid is a Toxin That Ought to be Banned

One other thing I want to bring up here, because I don't feel like it belongs in the food category, is folic acid. Folic acid is a by-product of the mining industry. It's been added to commercial wheat flours since 1998 in the US and since 2008 in Australia as it reduces the risk of neural tube defects in babies during early development (426; 427). For instance, research shows that its addition reduces spina bifida by 37%. That's a significant decrease (428).

But there's evidence it binds to folate receptors, preventing use of organic folate and impairing methylation. It's linked to inflammation and autoimmune disease through its effects on gene expression (429; 430).

Aside from decreasing your ability to properly regulate gene expression, it can also cause a rise in homocysteine. Homocysteine is an amino acid derived from methionine; an amino acid found in many foods. It contributes to oxidative stress through two key mechanisms.

First, homocysteine auto-oxidizes. It reacts with oxygen, forming ROS like hydrogen peroxide and superoxide radicals. These ROS are highly reactive. They can damage lipids, proteins, and DNA. This contributes to oxidative stress in the body (431).

Secondly, high homocysteine levels inhibit antioxidant enzyme activity. For example, homocysteine can impair superoxide dismutase and glutathione peroxidase. These enzymes are crucial for neutralising ROS and maintaining redox balance (432).

Moreover, homocysteine disrupts nitric oxide (NO), which is a vasodilator. It is vital for blood vessel health. This interference can cause endothelial dysfunction. It reduces the body's ability to manage oxidative stress. This is linked to outcomes like cardiovascular disease, hypertension, autoimmune disease, and especially Raynaud's (433; 434).

For people with methylenetetrahydrofolate reductase (MTHFR) gene mutations in particular, this can be a problem. They already have impaired folate methylation. For instance, folic acid supplements in pregnancy may contribute to allergies and autism in kids (435; 436). In adults, a faulty methylation pathway is linked to chronic inflammation and autoimmune diseases (437). I'm not talking about a small number of people here either. In North America, Europe, and Australia, 10-20% of people have two copies (homozygous) of the C677T MTHFR polymorphism (including myself). This impairs their ability to methylate folate by a whopping 70% (438). Add folic acid into the mix and the consequences may well be disastrous.

As far as I'm concerned, it should be banned as a food additive and anyone looking to conceive should be advised instead to take a supplement with a bioavailable form of folate – or to concentrate on getting more foods that contain it into their diet.

If you have MTHFR or other methylation polymorphisms, avoid this toxin. It will do more harm than good. Even if you don't, getting natural folate will help. It will make it easier for your body to detoxify and reduce inflammation. In countries with mandatory folic acid fortification, buy organic grain products. That's the only way to avoid folic acid in your diet unless you avoid grains completely.

I recommend researching your country's folic acid policy. It will show you what to avoid.

Are Pathogens Triggering Your Immune Response?

We've all been sick from some sort of pathogen at some time in the past. Things like the common cold, the flu, and yes, COVID-19 are all caused by viruses, a form of pathogen.

When you get a viral infection, it's usually minor. Your immune system should handle it quickly. Then, it should return to balance. But, if it's a nasty bout of something, it can cause chronic immune activation. If the immune system is under strain and lacks the resources to cope, this situation can occur. Or it can occur if the response needed is so high it shocks the system into overdrive. Recent research found that COVID-19 raises the risk of autoimmune disease by 43% (439). It is likely due to COVID's induction of acute inflammation, which compounds pre-existing low-grade inflammation. This may tip the immune system, causing autoimmune diseases and other post-COVID issues (440).

You likely know how to reduce your risk of contagious infections like COVID-19. There will be more research on this. But research shows that the best long-term strategy is to reduce its severity. This can be done by having a healthy immune system before infection. This means having a healthy redox balance (441; 442). You already know how to do that: reduce oxidative stress. So, if you've applied what you've learned in this book, you'll do much better. If you have long COVID, then what you've learned should also help manage or reverse your symptoms.

Persistent infections, such as mould and bacteria, may require something different. I see a lot of clients with mould and bacterial issues (443). They've often jumped through every other medical hoop, hoping to get a diagnosis for their symptoms. But they were told there is nothing wrong with them. The big flags are for people with gut health issues. They often feel nauseous after eating, especially certain foods and have ongoing allergies and sinus problems. I've created a table of the most common complaints related to them. They mostly differ from those linked to autoimmune disease.

Mould	Bacteria
Bloating, gas, diarrhoea, constipation, and abdominal pain (444)	Bloating, gas, diarrhoea, constipation, and abdominal pain (445)
Intense cravings for sugary foods and refined carbohydrates (446)	Unintentional weight loss and nutrient deficiencies, such as vitamin B12 deficiency, which can lead to anaemia and other related symptoms (447)
Frequent sinus infections, ear infections, or urinary tract infections (448)	Frequent nausea, particularly after meals (449)
White patches on the tongue and inside of the mouth (450)	Increased sensitivity to certain foods, especially those high in carbohydrates and fibre (although not limited to these foods) (447)

If you have any of these symptoms, get a faecal analysis. It's the best way to diagnose a bacterial or fungal infection. If you suspect mould issues, a urinary mycotoxin test may be helpful. These are the toxins produced by mould. Please note that a colonoscopy is unlikely to pick either of these up. Faeces and urine are the most effective diagnostic tools.

I also have a microscope that I use to check blood samples for parasites. This is only relevant if someone has or has had leaky gut and the parasites have escaped into the bloodstream but it's still a great tool. And hint: many of you will have leaky gut.

I would also suggest working with a clinician. These infections can be tricky and if they last a long time, the pathogens may have taken hold. They can take a long time to overcome. Because bacteria can make you nauseous every time you eat something they don't like, you might be missing out on micronutrients needed to nourish yourself and your good gut bacteria. An experienced clinician will be able to guide you through the process of getting rid of them and support you along the way.

If you have mould in your house or workplace, it's likely a source of gut issues. Eliminate it. But avoid using harmful chemicals. Appeal to the company you work for if you're not self-employed and it's in your workplace. If you're renting and it's at home, it should be up to your landlord/agent to organise its removal.

Bacterial gut infections can come from any number of sources. It can come from contaminated food or drink. But a diet can also allow harmful bacteria to thrive over those linked to better health. The best strategy is through diet, herbs, and persistence. But please make sure you're supported by someone who can guide you through the process.

You can also add more fermented foods or a diverse probiotic to your diet. This may help balance your gut microbiome. If your gut health isn't too impaired, this may help. It could reduce harmful, overgrown microbes (451; 452). But, it's important to monitor how you feel when you take probiotics or ferments. They can also make things worse in some instances.

Things to Include in Your Environment

So far in this section, I've spent a lot of time talking about things to avoid. Time now to talk about the things that you need to have more of in your environment to optimise your health.

Let's start with talking about temperature. Temperature tends to be a divisive issue for those with autoimmune diseases. You're either way too hot or way too cold.

Heat Therapy and Raynaud's

I fall into the latter camp. My toes and fingers are often numb. There's a reason for this, which is somewhat, but not entirely, outside my control. I have polymorphisms in my nitric oxide synthase (NOS3) gene that predisposes me to often feeling cold.

Remember how protein is good for nitric oxide (NO) production? NOS3 genes produce NO. If you have my genes, you're more likely to have poor vasodilation. That means your body has to work harder to get enough warm blood to your extremities in the cold.

NOS3 is linked to Raynaud's, a condition often co-morbid with autoimmune diseases (453; 454). You can still get Raynaud's even without my mutations, or any others linked to NOS3 issues. Oxidative stress reduces our body's ability to produce NOS3, via several mechanisms. It's an energetically expensive process, so when mitochondrial function is impaired, our body has to prioritise how it uses energy. ROS can also damage the NOS3 enzyme, as well as degrade NO itself. There can also be less of the substrates used to make NO available.

With Raynaud's, you're experiencing vasoconstriction, a narrowing of your blood vessels. It prevents blood from pumping through the blood vessels, especially to your extremities. The results are any or all of the following symptoms (455; 456).

- The skin changes colour (turning white when cold, blue as oxygen in the blood is depleted, and red when blood flow returns).
- Numbness or tingling in outer extremities, followed by cold.
- Mild swelling once blood flow is restored.
- Pain or discomfort when blood flow is restored.
- Smooth or tight skin.
- Ulcers and sores (in more extreme cases).

Aside from eating protein, which we've covered, and reducing stress, heat therapy is one of the best ways to boost NO production. I love the feeling of being warm. As a child, I loved to lie on the hot rock at my favourite beach. I would let the sun's heat seep in from both sides. Now I know that I probably loved it so much because it was working wonders for my NO production.

If you're keen to see if heat therapy helps you, try having saunas or hot baths regularly. Studies suggest sauna sessions at 80-100°C (176-212°F) for 10-20 minutes, followed by a cool-down, can greatly increase NO production, improve heart function, and boost well-being. It is recommended to repeat this process 2-3 times per week. Heat exposure causes vasodilation and boosts blood flow. It stimulates NO release, which improves endothelial function and reduces inflammation (457; 458).

You can also try a red-light sauna. The temperature can be a little lower for this (38-50°C/100.4-122°F), but it's just as effective. Try 20-30 minutes a few times per week (459).

It may sound expensive, but many gyms have saunas now. You can get two for the price of one.

Cold Therapy
Cold therapy may not be appropriate for you if you often feel cold. I hate the thought of plunging myself into ice-cold water. Why? It's very beneficial for many. It constricts your blood vessels, as low NO production does. For me, it's exacerbating what's already naturally taking place in my body.

For others, it can act as a hormetic stressor and improve NO production. But if the thought of it terrifies you, safe to say it's a little too stressful for your body to handle right now. If not, read on.

Ice baths have become popular in the last couple of years due to the work of one man, Wim Hoff, aka "Ice Man". He credits his amazing athleticism, endurance, and immunity to ice baths and his breathing technique, known as polycyclic breathing (460).

I won't discuss polycyclic breathing. I don't recommend it for everyone with an autoimmune disease, though you can look it up by googling him if you're interested. Please note, if you do try it, do it in the morning to avoid disrupting your circadian rhythm (more on this later). Also, your immune overactivity may trigger your immune system. Monitor how you feel afterwards, and if you feel worse, don't try it again until your immune system is more stable.

On the subject of ice baths, there are a couple of points I want to make. First, you don't have to get into an ice bath to get some of the benefits of it. A 2010 study showed that immersing your face in cold (14°C or 57.2°F) water for 30 seconds while holding your breath, then resting for 1-2 minutes, is just as effective for improving vagus nerve function. Repeat this. Do this a few times. Your ANS will likely become more parasympathetic dominant, helping to regulate your immune system (461).

You can also try contrast hydrotherapy. It involves alternating between hot and cold. 30 seconds of cold, 2 minutes of hot a few times can reportedly work wonders. It stimulates your lymphatic system, helping remove ROS and improving circulation. The result is less inflammation and pain. It's a gentler option for people, especially those with Raynaud's who dislike full-body immersion (462; 463). Make sure to do this in the morning though, not at night, as it may disrupt your sleep.

To get the full benefits of cold therapy, you must dunk your whole body. It will develop and stimulate brown fat. It's called "brown" because it has energy-burning mitochondria, like muscle. BUT, it doesn't have to be ice cold. If you're biologically female or new to cold exposure, it may be too stressful for you. Instead, try 16°C (60.8°F) water and see how you go with that. You may be able to gradually decrease the temperature to ice cold over time (464). If you can't or don't want to get to that point, that's fine. Or if you notice you feel worse afterwards, rather than energised, don't worry about it – it may not be the right thing for you. Go spend some time in the sauna instead.

The literature recommends 1-3 times a week for 10-15 minutes, though this varies a lot between individuals (462; 465). Again, I would encourage you to track how you feel. If you feel fantastic afterwards, keep it up and push yourself a little more next time. If not, back it off and go easy on yourself.

Your Aesthetic Environment
This section wouldn't be complete without discussing environmental aesthetics. This is an often overlooked but vital part of healing from an autoimmune disease. I could write a whole book about why this is so important but I'm going to keep things short and to the point here.

Until quite recently, humans lived in nature. It has many forms, sounds, smells, and tastes, but one of the defining characteristics of natural environments is the presence of fractal patterns (466). These are repeating patterns. Research suggests that we may think in fractal patterns, though this is yet to be confirmed (467). What we do know is that sensory exposure to fractal patterns seems to modulate the nervous system, bringing a sense of calm accompanied by a decrease in inflammatory biomarkers (468; 469). For most people, being in nature is an instant panacea for many of the things that ail them.

I noticed this when I first started to get sick with Hashimoto's. It felt like a relief every time I drove out of the city, leaving the traffic and bright lights behind. Two days in the country always had me feeling energised again. I felt as though I had come back to myself. But I always felt a pang as I headed back to the city: a physiological protest against returning to the concrete jungle I lived in.

My research on time in nature found it can reset your nervous system. The city's constant stimulation puts our sympathetic nervous system into overdrive. Our body interprets all the noise, light, and constant bustle as a threat. Even looking at streetscapes can bring you stress (470).

Spending as little as a few minutes in nature can restore our parasympathetic nervous system. Fresh air and natural views help as well. And guess what?

The more time you spend in nature, the more benefits you get from spending time in nature.

There's no point in going out there with your phone. You'll just end up watching cat videos on Instagram. The key to it is to be present and immersed in the experience. Let yourself be enchanted and mesmerised by the world around you. Take in as much sensory information as possible. If you do take your phone, make sure to leave it on aeroplane mode, so it doesn't interrupt the experience.

If you can't easily reach a natural area, try city parks. If you live in a leafy area with birds, that helps too. Again, paying attention to the sights and sounds around you is key (471). We have a magpie (a type of Australian bird) couple that regularly come up to our house. We've been feeding them for a couple of years now and have had the privilege of meeting two of their babies. It's a small thing, to have them eat from our hands a few times a week. But the wonder and joy it brings lifts my mood all day.

Harsh white light and clutter are two things that bug me. I have sensory processing issues, which means that I struggle with sensory overload. We've changed all the light bulbs to dim warm light, which I believe is what everyone should have in their homes and offices anyway. Clutter I can't stand either. It's not just that it can make things hard to find. I find it hard to *look at*.

I LOVE to have art, colours that match, and soft furnishings in my space. These things might not move you, but if they do – pay attention. There's nothing wrong with wanting nice things or being picky about your environment. Studies show that a pleasing environment can reduce stress and improve wellbeing (472; 473). Aesthetics do this by reducing sympathetic activation whilst increasing parasympathetic activity.

Your environment's aesthetics are not just a matter of preference. They reflect your relationship with the world and, by extension, yourself. Embracing nature, by spending time outdoors or creating a calming space at home, is an act of self-care. It reminds us that we are part of a web of life. Nurturing that connection is vital for our well-being.

Activity

For this activity, you're going to do an audit of your immediate environment. This can include just your household, though I recommend extending it to your street and your neighbourhood. The first thing to do is walk around the house and make a list (or a pile!) of any synthetic products that may potentially be contributing to oxidative stress.

Over the coming days and weeks, your mission is to replace anything on this list with products that don't contain substances that you now know are endocrine disruptors. When you seek a replacement, make sure to read the labels of everything so you're not being sold something just as bad or worse that's labelled "natural". You have your list of problem substances, so take it with you to shops if need be.

I also want you to take a good look at your house. Is there any mould that you can see anywhere? If there is, how pervasive is it? Can you remove it through cleaning? If not, it may be worth calling in a professional to help.

Ask yourself the following questions as well.

1. What is the temperature of my house like *for me?* Am I constantly too cold or too hot? Is there anything I can do to adjust the temperature to my preferences? AND should I be doing heat or cold therapy?
2. Does it make me feel happy when I come home? Is my home visually appealing to me? If not, what can I do to improve it?

Chapter Summary

- Environmental toxins are linked to various conditions, including cancer and autoimmune diseases.
- These toxins can interact with the immune system and genes, influencing autoimmune disease pathogenesis through various mechanisms such as immune suppression, gene activation, and oxidative stress.
- Chemicals, including endocrine disruptors, are ubiquitous in personal care products, cleaning agents, food, air, and even rain.
- Endocrine disruptors, like BPA and phthalates, increase oxidative stress by generating reactive oxygen species (ROS) and impairing antioxidant defences, leading to DNA damage and inflammation.
- Household items, including synthetic cleaning products, can harm your microbiome and overall health; switching to natural alternatives is recommended.
- The "hygiene hypothesis" suggests that excessive cleanliness may increase susceptibility to autoimmune and allergic diseases due to a lack of microbial exposure.
- Personal care products may contain harmful endocrine disruptors like phthalates, parabens, and triclosan; choosing natural or low-tox brands can reduce exposure.

- Chemicals in food, especially glyphosate, pose potential health risks, including cancer and DNA damage.
- Glyphosate, widely used in agriculture, has been linked to cancer, oxidative stress, and other health issues, raising concerns about its safety despite regulatory approval.
- The Johnson case in 2018 highlighted the carcinogenic potential of glyphosate and corporate malfeasance in hiding its dangers, leading to significant legal repercussions.
- Despite legal and scientific challenges, glyphosate remains legal in many countries, leaving consumers to bear the responsibility for reducing exposure through mindful purchasing decisions.
- Folic acid is a synthetic form of folate mandated in US and Australian wheat flour to prevent neural tube defects.
- Folic acid reduces spina bifida by ~37% but can impair methylation, leading to inflammation and autoimmune issues by blocking use of organic folate, especially in those with MTHFR gene mutations.
- Elevated homocysteine associated with poor methylation contributes to oxidative stress and cardiovascular issues.
- Viral infections can trigger chronic immune activation and autoimmune diseases.
- COVID-19 increases the risk of autoimmune conditions due to heightened inflammation.
- Maintaining immune health and reducing oxidative stress can mitigate infection effects.

- Persistent mould and bacterial infections cause symptoms like digestive issues and nutrient deficiencies.
- Faecal and urinary mycotoxin analyses are effective for diagnosis.
- Addressing mould in living/work spaces and adjusting diet are crucial for recovery. Probiotics and fermented foods may improve mild infections but monitor carefully and work with a professional for more complex cases.
- Heat therapy (e.g., sauna) boosts nitric oxide production and cardiovascular health and improve circulation and Raynaud's symptoms.
- Cold therapy may worsen conditions like Raynaud's; alternative methods like contrast hydrotherapy can be used.
- Natural settings help reduce stress and improve well-being.
- An aesthetically pleasing environment with soft lighting and minimal clutter enhances relaxation.
- Creating a soothing personal space and spending time in nature benefit mental and physical health.
- Hair mineral analysis may provide crucial insights into the role that heavy metals are playing in your autoimmune disease.

You Were Born to Move

"If you won't... one day you may not be able to."

Ido Portal

We all know that exercise is good for our health. We have heard it a thousand million times. You were probably urged to exercise by your school, the media, and your doctor. They all stressed the need to get out there and sweat.

Guess what? I'm going to tell you the same thing. Almost.

I will explain, first, why it's good to do some sport, lift weights, dance, or walk a lap every morning. You should also set bigger fitness goals. Second, I will explain why you must enjoy your movement. It can boost your cognition, genetic expression, and mitochondrial function. Also, very important is to know why you shouldn't *overdo* movement and how to recognise when you are.

What *Normally* Happens When You Exercise

Physical activity produces a stress response, most of the time in the best kind of way. It's a hormetic stressor, resulting in a positive adaptive response (474). For example, if you're training for a sporting event, some stress on your body in the form of exercise will help. A bit of exercise every day or two will make you fitter and better able to handle the challenges of exercise.

The energetic deficit that comes with exercising is one of the main ways by which we do this. When you exercise, you're expending extra energy. You're asking the mitochondria in your cells to produce more energy, faster, to meet the demands of your movement or exercise. As you already know, when you break down food molecules into ATP, you create RS as a byproduct. During exercise, the muscles use more oxygen. This raises the production of reactive species (RS). This is because the electron transport chain in mitochondria becomes more active. More electrons can leak and react with oxygen to form RS. To counteract the elevated RS, your body's antioxidant defence systems are activated.

In a healthy person with redox in balance, exercise boosts fitness by inducing positive changes. One way this occurs is through the production of new mitochondria. Exercise stimulates this process, called mitochondrial biogenesis, by increasing the expression of genes involved in mitochondrial replication and function.

Remember how the energetic deficit caused by fasting can lead to an increase in mitochondrial biogenesis? The same mechanism is at work here when you exercise. An energetic deficit activates these pathways, leading to more mitochondria. More mitochondria boost ATP production to meet higher energy demands. At the same time, more ATP-producing enzymes are made. The process becomes more efficient. With regular exercise, more ATP will be produced with less RS generation. This lowers oxidative stress and boosts the cell's energy capacity (475).

When Exercise Isn't Good for You

High oxidative stress can impair mitochondrial biogenesis through several mechanisms. First, high levels of RS and ROS can damage mitochondrial DNA (mtDNA). It's more prone to oxidative damage than nuclear DNA due to its proximity to the electron transport chain and limited repair mechanisms (476). This damage can impair the production of mitochondrial proteins, which mitochondria need to replicate and function.

Also, high oxidative stress can damage mitochondrial proteins and fats, affecting their structure and function. This damage disrupts the mitochondrial respiratory chain complexes, which are crucial for making ATP and creating new mitochondria (477).

As you now know, chronic oxidative stress causes inflammation. Inflammatory molecules like tumour necrosis factor alpha (TNF-α) and interleukin-6 (IL-6) can also harm mitochondria. They do this by blocking factors that regulate mitochondrial production and function (478). This inflammatory environment creates a feedback loop. Oxidative stress leads to inflammation, but inflammation can lead to oxidative stress. Both also hinder mitochondrial biogenesis by disrupting cellular energy balance. That becomes a problem because cells may prioritise survival over making new mitochondria (479). And then what happens? More energetic deficits, mitochondria working harder, more ROS production and oxidative stress, and then more immune activity. And so the cycle continues.

How Exercise Impacts the Antioxidant Defence System

Exercise has a considerable impact on your antioxidant defence system via changing nervous system activity. When you exercise, the sympathetic nervous system (SNS) is activated. This activation raises heart rate and blood pressure and also redirects blood flow to the working muscles. It ensures more oxygen and nutrients reach the muscles to meet their higher energy demands (480). During exercise, the parasympathetic nervous system (PNS) is less active. But, after exercise, the PNS helps the body recover by becoming more active again.

A crucial aspect of the PNS's activity involves the upregulation of antioxidant systems. For example, increased superoxide dismutase (SOD) activity converts superoxide radicals into less harmful hydrogen peroxide and oxygen. PNS activation boosts SOD activity (481). Similarly, glutathione peroxidase (GPx) and catalase break down hydrogen peroxide into water and oxygen. This prevents oxidative damage to cells. Their levels rise after exercise due to PNS stimulation (482; 483).

The PNS also supports glutathione (GSH) production (which we talked about in the section on diet) and recycling. GSH scavenges ROS and maintains redox balance by neutralising ROS (484). Like all antioxidants, it works closely with the lymphatic system to remove waste and debris from tissues. Guess what? Increased PNS activity stimulates lymphatic flow. Meanwhile, having extra GSH floating around helps move substrates to the lymphatic system for removal. Their combined effects support cell health and recovery after exercise.

Additionally, post-exercise PNS modulation reduces heart rate, promoting digestion and recovery (480). It also stimulates the release of neurotransmitters such as norepinephrine, dopamine, and serotonin. These neurotransmitters play a dual role in boosting mood, focus, and alertness and helping balance the SNS and PNS (485).

But, in those with autoimmune diseases, chronic oxidative stress may keep the SNS *overly* active. As I outlined, exercise causes acute inflammation as the body adapts. More SNS stimulation from exercise can worsen symptoms like fatigue, pain, and cognitive dysfunction (486). This is because the immune system becomes activated even more (487). Also, PNS activity may be impaired. This can lead to poor recovery from exercise and may cause long-lasting fatigue, sore muscles, and a higher risk of injuries and infections (488).

In 2018, I learned that too much or the wrong exercise worsens autoimmune disease. I've been a long-distance runner for most of my life and usually feel exhilarated and energised after a run. After I got sick with Hashimoto's, I lacked the energy to run as fast or as far as I used to. I also felt *worse* after a run. Plus, the more I exercised, the more weight I seemed to put on. I took a while to admit it to myself. But, I had to face the fact that, at that point in my life, the exercise I had always done and loved wasn't good for me.

Learn from my mistake. If you feel sore and achy after you exercise, then you're likely pushing yourself too hard. *Chill.*

This raises the question: *what exercise should you do with an autoimmune disease?*

The answer is nuanced. You must do something that is good for you and that you enjoy, so it's sustainable in the long term. Don't start something just because you feel you have to. It's only going to create more stress for you.

In saying that, there's no harm in trying a few different forms of exercise until you find one that fits. When choosing what to do, there are a couple of core principles that are worth keeping in mind.

Weight-Bearing Exercise

Weight-bearing exercises, like resistance training and weightlifting, are vital for physical health. They improve many aspects of it. This is especially true for those with autoimmune conditions. These exercises stress the bones and muscles. This triggers beneficial changes in the body.

Weight-bearing exercises have been shown to help those with rheumatoid arthritis. They improve muscle strength around inflamed, damaged joints. This increased strength supports the joints while also reducing pain and improving function (489).

Furthermore, weight-bearing exercises contribute to the maintenance and improvement of bone density. This is vital. Autoimmune diseases and drugs used to manage them, like corticosteroids, can cause bone loss and raise osteoporosis risk. These exercises stimulate bone growth and remodelling. Weight-bearing exercises help mitigate the negative effects on bone health (490).

Physical function is also enhanced through regular weight-bearing exercises. It increases balance, coordination, and flexibility, all vital for daily activities and quality of life. Weight-bearing exercises can help manage symptoms and maintain daily independence (489; 490).

Additionally, increased muscle tone contributes to better regulation of blood pressure. As previously discussed, many people with autoimmune diseases have issues with blood pressure being too high or too low. Some researchers now see hypertension and postural tachycardia syndrome (POTS) as autoimmune diseases in and of themselves, which I think in some instances may be correct (491; 492).

Weight-bearing exercises can help in the management of blood pressure via several mechanisms. Muscles regulate blood flow and vascular tone, improving vasodilation. When muscles contract during exercise, they release vasodilators like nitric oxide (NO). This dilation of blood vessels increases blood flow and reduces resistance, lowering blood pressure.

Additionally, regular exercise improves cardiovascular fitness. This includes muscle-toning activities like resistance training. These kinds of activities strengthen the heart muscle, so it pumps blood more efficiently with each beat. A stronger heart can pump more blood per beat, which can help to lower blood pressure over time.

Muscle contractions during exercise help move blood to active muscles from inactive areas. This redistribution of blood reduces resistance in blood vessels. This is a key factor in blood pressure. Lower resistance means the heart doesn't have to work as hard to circulate blood, resulting in lower overall blood pressure (493).

Weight-bearing exercises also offer the benefits of exercise with less risk of increasing sympathetic nervous system (SNS) dominance. Cardiovascular stress can raise SNS activity and lowers PNS influence to increase heart rate. However, excessive SNS activity can trigger a higher immune response, increase ROS production, and hinder recovery (489; 490). Also, high SNS activity can raise blood pressure. So, weight-bearing exercises are safer compared to cardiovascular exercises for people with autoimmune conditions.

To do weight-bearing exercises well, focus on two things. First, get your technique right. Second, apply progressive overload. Use bigger, compound movements, like squats and deadlifts. They are better than smaller, single-muscle exercises. They will give you more from your weighted workouts. You can also use bodyweight exercises at first. If you find compound movements hard with weights, then gradually add some weight once you're confident. It will let you perfect your technique. This reduces the risk of injury while you learn the movements.

Another hack if you're doing weight training in a gym environment is to use machines. Because of the way that they're designed, it's so much easier (though not impossible!) to complete a movement with good technique, especially without a trainer or anyone to spot you and correct your form. No, you won't get quite the same benefits as if you were using free weights, but you will have less risk of injury.

Many YouTube channels show how to do these exercises well. If you can't afford a gym or a trainer, this is a great way to start weight training. You don't need to do weight training every day either – as little as a couple of sessions per week can yield benefits.

High-Intensity Interval Training

That said, if you want to do some cardio, there are smart ways to reduce the risk of high oxidative stress. The best way to do cardio with less risk of oxidative stress is high intensity interval training, or HIIT. BUT – I only recommend it if you're not in a flare-up and are starting to control your autoimmune condition. This means more good days than bad days and little or no regular joint pain.

HIIT is when we do intense activity for short bursts. We then rest before another bout of intense activity. The activity periods are shorter, so they produce less RS in total. This reduces the risk of an ANS imbalance. They also help the body recover and manage oxidative stress from the workout. But you still get all the benefits of exercise. These include a boosted antioxidant defence and improved energy from better oxidative phosphorylation.

HIIT workouts can boost metabolism significantly. In fact, they can burn the same amount of energy as longer endurance cardio workouts over 24 hours. This is despite being shorter and using less energy during the workout itself.

A 2014 study compared three groups: one that did a HIIT program, another that did 50 minutes of cardio, and one that didn't exercise. It found that the HIIT group had the same results as the cardio group in terms of energy expenditure. But they only did 10 minutes of exercise and less than half as much work (494).

But I want to make something very clear here. When I say HIIT, I don't mean those weird classes where you spend 45 minutes frantically going from one activity to the next, with no chance to catch your breath. I'm talking about short-duration work at a very high intensity.

For instance, a study found that two minutes of exercise three times a week for six weeks was enough to promote the same adaptations as 30 minutes of cardio three times a week for six weeks (495). With HIIT training, the key is to go hard during the work. Then, have a short recovery, but not so long that you need to warm up again. This way, you can go hard again in the next bout. A great way to start is with a warmup: jog, row, or cycle lightly for 3-7 minutes. Don't go so hard that you can't talk. Just go hard enough to breathe a bit faster.

In the high-intensity interval, give it your all. Use 80-90% of your max effort for 20-60 seconds. Then give yourself anywhere between 1-4 minutes to recover before doing the next bout. The recovery time should be lightly active, so you're not straining at all but keeping things moving. So, if your intervals are sprinting on foot, then walking slowly is perfect. If you're rowing or cycling, keep moving but slowly. It shouldn't hurt, and you should catch your breath. Repeat the interval & rest cycle anywhere between 3-10 times.

As you get more fit, you'll notice that you can go a little longer and need less recovery time between bouts. Keep on pushing yourself a little more as your body adapts, though don't push too far too fast. Give your body time to adapt before reducing recovery time, increasing bouts, or increasing the interval time. If you push too much too quickly, you're likely to increase oxidative stress again. And please don't do this more than two or three times a week. The recovery time between bouts is crucial for this type of exercise to yield its benefits.

If you take a long time to recover after HIIT and feel terrible, this is a sure sign that you're pushing yourself too hard. Stop doing it for a while. Wait until your symptoms have improved and your immune system is less active. Then, you can push yourself with HIIT. It will still be there when you've recovered enough for it to be beneficial.

Bonus tip: At the end of every workout, try slow, deep breathing. It helps your nervous system calm down and speeds up recovery (496).

Yoga, Pilates, And the OG Best Exercise for Humans: Walking

Yoga and Pilates are also great options for those with autoimmune diseases. I'm no expert on either. However, I know of excellent research showing that they improve outcomes in people with autoimmune diseases. A 2021 study looked at mitochondrial health in people with rheumatoid arthritis before and after an 8-week yoga program. This was an intensive intervention, where the participants practised yoga for 120 minutes five times a week. Unfortunately, the study didn't specify a type of yoga, but it did mention that it included postures, breathing, and meditation. It found that yoga improved and optimized various markers of mitochondrial health, as well as circadian rhythm (497).

Meanwhile, Pilates has improved function in people with Multiple Sclerosis. It helped their balance, coordination, strength, and cognition (498).

Even regular walking can help those with autoimmune diseases. Walking is a low-impact exercise, so it's gentle on sore joints and muscles while keeping joints flexible and easing stiffness and pain (499). In women with Sjogren's syndrome, walking improved fitness and reduced fatigue (500). A study last year found that walking can improve sleep and quality of life in lupus patients (501). These combined benefits highlight the value of walking. It can improve the physical and mental well-being of those with autoimmune diseases.

Make it Fun

No matter what exercise you do, it's important to do it. Do it consistently. And give your body small amounts of progressive overload without pushing too hard. A recent review article found exercise helps people with autoimmune diseases so long as whatever you do suits *your* individual needs (502). Focus on what feels good for you, what's achievable, and what you enjoy.

Choose activities that fulfil your needs and preferences. This includes weight-bearing exercises, HIIT, yoga, or walking. Any or all of these have the potential to be beneficial. Listen to your body and avoid overexertion. By doing so, you not only enhance your current health but also protect your future mobility.

Choose fun, mindful exercises today. They will keep you moving and thriving in the future. Embrace movement now to preserve your freedom and vitality for years to come.

Challenge

If you're not already active in some way, I'd love to challenge you to be more active. But I don't want you to push yourself too far outside your comfort zone. I want you to find the *smallest* possible physical activity you can do. It needs to be something you're not already doing. It also needs to be something that doesn't feel so uncomfortable you dread it.

If you're not active at all right now, you could try stretching for five minutes in the morning. A walk around the block. Ten minutes of yoga. Whatever feels safe and comfortable. I want you to commit to doing this at least three times per week for the next month. And then I want you to write down how you feel afterwards. It doesn't have to be much, just a few descriptive words. Enough so that you will be able to look back and understand what exercise does for you.

If you're coming up with words like "exhausted", "tired", or "pain", then that's also a pretty good sign to back it off a bit. But if your words are "relaxed", "invigorated", or "happy" then you know you're onto a good thing.

Chapter Summary

- Exercise is widely acknowledged for its health benefits and is encouraged by various sources including schools, media, and health professionals.
- Engaging in physical activities like sports, weight lifting, dancing, or walking can improve fitness, cognitive function, genetic expression, and mitochondrial health.
- Exercise acts as a hormetic stressor, promoting positive adaptations such as increased fitness and mitochondrial biogenesis, which enhances energy production and reduces oxidative stress.
- Overdoing exercise can lead to excessive oxidative stress, damaging mitochondrial DNA and proteins, disrupting key signalling pathways (AMPK, PGC-1α), and exacerbating inflammation.
- Regular exercise activates the sympathetic nervous system (SNS) during activity and the parasympathetic nervous system (PNS) post-exercise, which aids in recovery and supports antioxidant systems.
- Individuals with autoimmune diseases may experience worsened symptoms from exercise due to pre-existing oxidative stress and immune dysregulation.
- Weight-bearing exercises improve muscle strength, bone density, and overall physical function, which is beneficial for those with autoimmune conditions.
- High-intensity interval training (HIIT) can be effective if managed carefully, allowing for high

energy expenditure with less risk of oxidative stress compared to continuous cardio.

- Yoga and Pilates offer significant benefits for autoimmune disease management, including improved mitochondrial health, balance, and coordination.
- Regular walking provides a low-impact exercise option that can enhance joint flexibility, cardiovascular fitness, and overall well-being for those with autoimmune conditions.
- It's essential to choose enjoyable and suitable forms of exercise, progressively increasing intensity while avoiding overexertion to ensure long-term health and mobility.

Inadequate Sleep is More Than Just Mental Torture

"Sleep is the golden chain that ties health and our bodies together."

Thomas Dekker

Sleep is vital, but often overlooked, for managing autoimmune diseases and the immune system. It's something that I have struggled with for most of my life. Right before I developed Hashimoto's, my sleep was terrible. I would sometimes get as little as three hours a night. In the last few years, I've finally learned how to get good sleep, consistently.

I don't think I'm alone in this. Many of us seem to have real problems with getting enough high-quality sleep. We'll discuss good sleep and how to get it shortly. But first, let's talk about sleep's role in your health because it's especially important for those with autoimmune diseases.

The role of sleep itself has puzzled researchers for a long time, but it's clearly important. In 1989, researchers sleep-deprived 10 rats to study the effects. Unfortunately for the poor rats, they all died or were put down within 11-32 days. The sleep-deprived rats "looked sickly, had tail and paw lesions, and lost weight despite eating more." The mechanism of debilitation and weight loss in the rats seems to be increased energy expenditure. This was consistent across all the rats (503).

You might suspect why increased energy use hurt the rats. It likely resulted in an increase in oxidative stress, albeit via a roundabout route. To see how it might raise oxidative stress, let's first examine how it boosts energy use.

The Effects of Sleep Deprivation on Oxidative Stress

Sleep deprivation increases energy use through several mechanisms. These involve hormonal regulation, a higher metabolic rate, and changes in the sympathetic nervous system.

Hormonal dysregulation, with lower leptin and higher ghrelin, led to increased food intake and a higher metabolic rate to process the extra energy (504). Leptin is a hormone that signals fullness. Ghrelin is a hormone that triggers hunger.

Ghrelin primarily comes from the stomach. We're still getting our heads around how exactly its production is initiated, but your gut microbiota likely helps produce it. So do inflammatory cytokines like interleukin 6 (IL-6) and tumour necrosis factor-alpha (TNF-a) (505; 506). When you're awake, you use more energy than when asleep. Even doing a sedentary activity burns fuel faster. So, your gut will produce more ghrelin to compensate. Meanwhile, sleep-wake cycles and circadian rhythms reduce leptin production in fat tissues. This allows ghrelin to raise appetite, increasing food intake (507).

Sleep deprivation also leads to elevated cortisol levels. As we've discussed, cortisol boosts metabolic rate by activating the SNS. This raises heart rate and blood pressure, increasing energy use (508). Cortisol also promotes gluconeogenesis, a process that breaks down non-carb macronutrients, like amino acids and glycerol (a key component of fats), for fuel. This ensures enough glucose to meet the body's energy needs during stress. However, faster metabolism and increased glucose production create more reactive species (RS). If the body's antioxidants can't manage them, they cause damage and stress (318). High glucose and RS can also cause insulin resistance and risk of type 2 diabetes, as well as other metabolic disorders. They, in turn, raise the risk of autoimmune disease (507; 509).

Thermogenesis also plays a role in increased energy use during sleep deprivation. This process involves producing heat in brown fat tissue (BAT) to help the body stay balanced. BAT is unique because it burns energy to produce heat. This is due to a protein called UCP1 in its cells (510). We touched on this briefly in the discussion on cold therapy.

Lack of sleep raises hormones like norepinephrine, which activates BAT. It's involved in the stress response. The activation of norepinephrine is an adaptive response; it increases your body's metabolic rate and heat production to keep you warm (511). At the same time, extra energy use for thermoregulation adds to the stress on the body during times of not getting enough sleep.

Also, when you're sleep-deprived, you get more restless. You move around more, even if it's just fidgeting, which also raises your energy use (512).

These combined mechanisms increase the metabolic rate and energy use, which increases the RS load on the body, nudging the dial towards oxidative stress.

There's one other thing to note, though: sleep deprivation also compromises your antioxidant defence system.

Sleep is one of the rare times during the day when your ability to remove RS exceeds its production (513). Two factors play into this. Firstly, your basal metabolic rate is lower during sleep. RS production slows significantly. But also, your circadian rhythm is disrupted. Circadian rhythms control many biological processes, including antioxidant production and cellular repair. Lack of sleep disrupts these rhythms and reduces your body's ability to produce antioxidants and repair itself. This impairment means the body can't repair oxidative damage, leading to a buildup of damage and increased oxidative stress over time (514).

There are many other things that sleep, and sleep deprivation do, some of which we've touched one already. For example, rapid eye movement (REM) sleep helps with memory consolidation and moving on from trauma, which we discussed back in the chapter on emotional stress. A whole book is needed to go through them all. But I hope you get the point: sleep is essential. It slows the metabolism, produces antioxidants, repairs daily cellular damage, and maintains a healthy redox balance. What I'd like to do now is go through how we define as good sleep and how you can achieve it.

Based on the research, I've come up with six key markers for good sleep, as outlined in the sections below.

Adequate Duration

Adults need 7-9 hours of sleep per night for peak performance. This is according to the Sleep Health Foundation (515). Many studies link inadequate sleep to health issues. They include cognitive impairment, mood issues, and a higher risk of chronic diseases like hypertension and diabetes (516). However, sleep needs vary by genetics, age, health, and lifestyle (517). The more oxidative stress you're subject to, the more sleep you need. If you have an autoimmune disease, sleep is vital. You may need more than the guidelines.

Sleep duration and quality can be affected by many factors. These include physical activity, work schedules (especially shift work), and pre-sleep activities, like screen time (518). Poor sleep hygiene, like irregular sleep patterns and too much caffeine close to bedtime, worsens sleep and health risks (519). This may mean that you need to prioritise spending more time sleeping and/or in bed to get the same benefits of sleep.

Sleeping 7-9 hours minimum is the guideline, though you may need slightly more or slightly less than this. It's important to know and meet your sleep needs.

Sleep Continuity

Sleep should remain uninterrupted, allowing for few awakenings throughout the night. If you experience interruptions in your sleep, then it will be harder for you to reach the deep sleep stages. Parents of young children, I'm sure you know what I'm talking about.

Frequent awakenings at night disrupt sleep patterns. They reduce sleep quality. This disruption can cause fatigue, poor focus, and mood swings. Poor sleep continuity also links to insomnia, sleep apnoea, and other disorders. I'm sure you know this without me saying it: these are tied to increased oxidative stress-related conditions, including cardiovascular and metabolic diseases (520).

I suggest two main strategies to counter frequent sleep interruptions. Firstly, make sure that you sleep in an environment where you're less likely to have your sleep disrupted. This means the right temperature on your outer extremities. It should not be too hot or too cold – the optimal temperature range is 15.6-19.4°C or 60-67F (521). The room should be dark. Blackout curtains are great for this. It should be quiet. I used ear plugs for years in the city.

I understand that if you have kids or pets, getting a full night's sleep can be tricky. We always take our dog out at night to toilet him before bed. Still, he sometimes needs to go out, especially if he had water or a big meal before bed. We do what we can to mitigate this, but it doesn't always work. Do what you can.

Another thing that wakes many people, especially older folks, is waking up between 2-4am. They then find it hard to get back to sleep. There are a couple of reasons why people often wake up at night.

One of them is alcohol. I'm happy to go on record and say that I'm not anti-alcohol in general. In small amounts and at the right times, alcohol can facilitate social bonding (522). However, it's important you understand that alcohol has some serious side effects. One is higher cortisol levels. This rise in cortisol is linked to an activated HPA axis and more night wakings. It's not just the day you drink, either. Heavy drinking raises cortisol levels chronically. If you drink, keep it to a couple of drinks per week. If you get tipsy several times a week, it may disrupt your sleep and cause other issues that increase oxidative stress (523).

Low blood sugar is the other common culprit of early-morning wakefulness. This is called nocturnal hypoglycaemia (524). Cortisol is again involved here. Low blood sugar triggers cortisol release, promoting wakefulness, likely to get you to find food. To combat this, eat more protein in your pre-bed meal. Don't eat so much that it gives you "meat sweats" or makes your stomach gurgle all night. Try upping it slightly, by 5-10 grams of protein and see what that does for you. If you still find that you wake up, try adding a little more. Also, if you eat early, try eating a little later or having a high-protein snack before bed. Collagen is a great pre-bed protein. It also contains glycine, which improves sleep, because it acts as what's called an inhibitory neurotransmitter, calming your brain down. Take about 15 grams of collagen before bed or at the end of your night-time meal. It should do the trick (525).

Sleep Stages
It's important that you cycle through the different stages of sleep: light sleep, deep sleep, and rapid eye movement

(REM) sleep. Each plays a critical role in health and sleep's benefits.

Non-REM sleep is important because it's when the glymphatic system, the brain's waste removal system, is most active.

The body also releases the most growth hormone during this time (526; 527). This is important for cellular repair.

But REM sleep is also essential, as it seems to play a role in regulating the immune system. It acts like a check-in, letting the body assess its needs so it can make changes to reduce immune dysregulation (528). If you're not getting enough REM sleep, that check-in won't be happening. Your immune system may stay overactive, despite your best efforts.

We're also going to discuss the importance of sleep timing shortly, as it helps you maximize the different sleep stages. There's something else you can do, though. It's a bit counterintuitive to what we'll discuss in the timing section. It's to wake up without an alarm. I'm a huge fan of waking up naturally when my last REM cycle is complete. If you've ever woken from a vivid dream feeling disoriented and confused, it's probably because it was during your REM sleep cycle. If you let it finish and wake naturally, you'll wake more refreshed. And, because REM also acts as moderator of immune system activity, you'll also be less likely to experience autoimmune symptoms and flare ups.

This was a game changer for me when I was unwell with Hashimoto's. Even once I was back to working and supporting myself, I still didn't wake up with an alarm. I just let my body wake naturally.

Alcohol is another sleep cycle disruptor. It harms the processes in the different stages, especially REM sleep. Though it may help you sleep at first, it promotes cortisol and wakefulness later in sleep, reducing REM sleep. If you drink alcohol before bed, keep it to a minimum. Try to have it earlier in the night, not right before bedtime (529).

Exercise increases REM sleep duration (530). A study on people with rheumatoid arthritis found a 12-week, personalized exercise program improved sleep and reduced fatigue. Subjective reports also showed a significant reduction in pain and stiffness (531). Yet another reason for you to get some movement in each day.

Sleep Efficiency

Sleep efficiency is the ratio of time asleep to time in bed. It is calculated by dividing the total time asleep by the total time in bed, then multiplied by 100 to get a percentage. For example, if someone spends 8 hours in bed but only sleeps for 7 hours, their sleep efficiency would be 87.5%. That's 7 hours asleep divided by 8 hours in bed, times 100.

A high sleep efficiency, above 85%, is best. It means most of your time in bed is spent sleeping, not lying awake. This measure is important because it shows how well someone can sleep without interruption all night. It reflects the effectiveness of sleep consolidation. High sleep efficiency means better sleep quality and more restorative sleep, both of which are crucial for health and well-being (532; 533).

High sleep efficiency can be affected by many factors. They include sleep hygiene, regular sleep schedules, and treating sleep disorders. It is a key indicator in sleep medicine and is worth keeping track of if you have a wearable sleep tracker.

Timing

This is a big one many of us overlook. Keeping consistent sleep and wake times is crucial to good sleep. A consistent sleep schedule helps sync the circadian rhythm, which runs on a 24-hour cycle. It governs sleep-wake patterns, hormone secretion, and metabolism. The schedule aligns it with external cues, like light and darkness. This ensures optimal timing of physiological functions throughout the day and night (534).

A key benefit of consistent sleep times is the regulation of melatonin production. Melatonin is a hormone made by the pineal gland that promotes sleepiness and regulates the sleep-wake cycle. Regular sleep patterns teach the body when to release melatonin, helping you to fall asleep more easily and restfully (535). Also, a stable sleep schedule helps develop the proper sequence and duration of sleep stages, like REM and non-REM sleep, leading to deeper, more restorative sleep. This has been shown to improve sleep quality and daytime alertness (519).

Consistent sleep and wake times optimise other functions controlled by the circadian rhythm. These include hormone release, immune function, and metabolism (536). I want to highlight the role of consistent sleep timing in the release of growth hormone. Growth hormone secretion follows a pulsating pattern, with most secretion occurring during SWS or deep sleep. This usually happens earlier in the sleep cycle, so earlier in the night. Research suggests that regular sleep patterns support the body's natural hormone cycle, including growth hormone. Growth hormone is crucial for growth, metabolism, and tissue repair (537).

This is particularly important for autoimmune disease. You probably have some damage to organs and/or tissues due to antibody attacks, which GH has the potential to help your body heal. Also, evidence suggests that GH can modulate the immune response, possibly preventing autoimmune disease (538).

If you struggle to fall asleep, there are a couple of things you can try. First, do all the things you've heard elsewhere. Reduce blue light exposure before bed. Avoid doom-scrolling on your phone. Above all, avoid anything else that makes you feel alert (519).

You can also do things to actively promote relaxation. I love to take a warm bath before bed. I also listen to music, especially binaural beats in the delta wave frequency. Sometimes, I couple this with breathing exercises like box breathing. I try to avoid listening to a podcast or doing anything else that's stimulating and read a fiction book instead. You can also add essential oils, like lavender, to your bath to promote relaxation (so long as you don't have histamine intolerance or any other adverse reactions to them). It should go without saying, but also make sure to avoid synthetic fragrances.

One of my other favourite things to do is self-hypnotism. Yep, I know, it sounds scary. The truth is, it's anything but scary. I find it incredibly relaxing because it stops me from worrying about the future and things that haven't happened yet. I also feel less focused on the past and become more aware of my own body and the sensations I'm experiencing (539). It's a great way to make you fall asleep and can have lasting benefits for your nervous system (540).

I'm not trained to tell you how to do this, but if you're curious, I suggest you check out the REVERI app. It was designed by researchers from Stanford, Harvard, and Yale. They have a range of different self-hypnoses on there, including ones for sleep but also trauma processing (541).

If you're not quite ready to take on hypnosis, my other go-to is Yoga Nidra, which is not yoga as you know it. It's a series of interoceptive exercises sequenced to induce calm and, sometimes, sleep. My favourite recordings are from Kumari Sky, and they're available for free on Spotify. Search, and her recordings will come up, including some especially for sleep.

Another thing you can do is save your carbohydrates for nighttime (if you're eating carbs). We've already talked about how carbohydrates suppress cortisol production. It's normal to produce cortisol in the morning because it helps us wake up and gives us energy for the day. But cortisol production should taper off at night, and melatonin production should increase (542). If you're tired in the morning but wide awake at night, your circadian rhythm is off. Emphasising carbohydrates in your night meal should help reset your circadian rhythm.

Early morning sunlight also boosts cortisol, helping reset your circadian rhythm (543). If you do morning exercise outside, this can be a great way to get some sunlight in early on. Even sitting outside in the sun with your morning tea or coffee for 10 minutes can be helpful.

I know you're probably not going to want to hear this one but if you struggle to sleep, reducing your caffeine intake or even changing when you have it may also be helpful. Have it earlier in the day, decrease the amount you have, or cut it out completely. What's known as sleep pressure builds up during the day through the breakdown of ATP into adenosine. The more sleep pressure you have, the more tired you feel.

It works like this. Adenosine in the brain binds to specific adenosine receptors. This creates a greater sense of drowsiness as more adenosine builds up throughout the day from using energy. During sleep, adenosine is removed and either recycled or excreted. This promotes wakefulness once enough is removed from the receptors (544).

Caffeine helps you feel more alert by binding to adenosine receptors. This blocks adenosine from binding, creating a false sense of wakefulness, as caffeine doesn't interact with the receptors in the same way to make you sleepy (545; 546). The issue is that adenosine is intended to make you drowsy for a reason. For one thing, you've been utilising lots of energy, which has created lots of ROS and damage to cells. As you now know, you need sleep to repair cellular damage and remove ROS. If you rely on caffeine to stay awake, you don't simply remain awake. You're also more likely to cause higher oxidative stress. Your cells can't repair the damage, which will lead to more ROS production. If you're sleepy during the day, it's not a sign that you need more caffeine. It's a sign that you need to *sleep*.

One thing that I now do (when having coffee at home) is having a mostly decaf coffee with a little bit of caffeinated coffee. I'm lucky in that my partner works in the coffee industry, so I have access to truly delicious decaf (which I drink black), but there are more and more great decafs coming on the market. If you look, I'm pretty sure you'll find some good options. The little bit of caffeine doesn't affect how I feel all that much, I just like how the full-caffeine coffee adds a little bit more flavour and complexity.

Subjective Sense of Refreshment

At the end of the day, how refreshed and ready for the day you feel after a sleep is the most important aspect of good sleep. If you sleep eight or nine hours but feel awful when you wake up, something is wrong. You may need to change your sleep habits. If you've tried everything here and still see no improvement, it may be time to call a sleep specialist for help.

You can also try supplements. They can help you sleep and stay asleep. This will let you complete the proper sleep cycles. Here are some of my favourites.

Creatine

I know I've already mentioned creatine in this book, but I love it so much that I'm doing it again. It's one of my favourite supplements for sleep.

That said, the research on creatine's effects during sleep is still in its infancy: we don't know a lot about how it improves sleep. It reduces total sleep time but improves sleep quality, reducing the need for longer sleep duration. We're not exactly sure why, but a potential mechanism by which it does this is through the effects that it exerts on growth hormone production. We know that creatine boosts growth hormone production when taken after exercise. However, no research has studied its effects on growth hormone during sleep, so whether or not this is its mechanism of action is unclear (547).

Another possibility is its effects on GABA receptors. GABA is our brain's main inhibitory neurotransmitter. Creatine may act as an agonist and increase GABA production (548; 549). This research is still very much in its infancy, but it suggests that creatine may promote restfulness. Watch this space as research on creatine seems to have exploded recently. I don't think it will be long before we understand how it may promote sleep and better-quality sleep.

I sometimes take 5-10 grams of creatine monohydrate (the form I recommend) before bed. It seems to improve my sleep. But, who knows how much is placebo versus real effects? I started taking creatine for its GH production benefits. Within just a few short days, a whole heap of other benefits emerged. It reduced my brain fog and boosted my energy, likely because my methylation was so poor at the time and methylation plays a major role in creatine production. Better sleep is a nice side effect as well.

Magnesium

Magnesium is a crucial mineral that supports various bodily functions, including muscle and nerve activity, blood sugar regulation, and bone health. Magnesium regulates neurotransmitters like serotonin, which affects mood and sleep. It's also a natural muscle relaxant that calms the nervous system by enhancing GABA activity, helping to manage stress response (550). Low magnesium levels can disrupt the balance between alertness and relaxation, increasing stress and anxiety and leading to poor sleep (551). It also helps control cortisol, promoting relaxation and better sleep (552).

Magnesium supplementation has shown positive effects on sleep, especially in those with deficiencies or high stress. A clinical trial found magnesium improved sleep quality and reduced insomnia symptoms in the elderly (553). It also helps prevent muscle cramps that can disturb sleep (554) Common dietary sources include leafy greens, nuts, and seeds, but many people may need supplements, especially under stress (555).

I will place a caveat on this though, based on personal experience. People with excess serotonin due to certain genetic mutations may actually find magnesium detrimental to sleep. It may also be an issue for those with impaired kidney function as it's excreted by the kidneys. So, always pay attention to how you feel after starting to take it.

For sleep, the best magnesium forms are:

1. **Magnesium Glycinate**: Bound to glycine, this form promotes relaxation and improves sleep with minimal gastrointestinal side effects. Recommended dose: 200-400mg (556).
2. **Magnesium Citrate**: Highly bioavailable, it can aid sleep and ease occasional constipation as it has a mild laxative effect. Dose: 200-400mg (557).
3. **Magnesium Threonate**: Penetrates the blood-brain barrier, potentially enhancing cognitive function and sleep quality. Dose: 1000-2000mg spread throughout the day (558).
4. **Magnesium Taurate**: Combines magnesium with taurine, supporting cardiovascular health and calming the nervous system. Dose: 200-400mg (559).
5. **Magnesium Chloride**: Absorbs well and can be taken orally or used topically (e.g., magnesium oil). Oral dose: 200-400mg (560).

L-Theanine

L-Theanine is an amino acid in tea leaves, especially green tea. It promotes relaxation and improves sleep, but it doesn't cause drowsiness. It increases alpha brain waves, which produce relaxed alertness. This helps reduce stress and anxiety (561). L-theanine also boosts GABA, serotonin, and dopamine. They are key for mood, relaxation, and sleep (562). Additionally, it may lower cortisol, aiding stress reduction and better sleep (563).

Unlike sedatives, L-theanine relaxes without causing drowsiness. So, it's ideal for improving sleep without impairing alertness (564). It can shorten the time to fall asleep and increase sleep duration. This is especially true for those with anxiety or stress-related sleep issues (565). L-theanine, often combined with melatonin or magnesium, boosts their sleep effects (566).

Research supports L-theanine's effectiveness in improving sleep quality. For example, Lyon et al. (564) found it improved sleep efficiency in boys with ADHD, although I would take this finding with a pinch of salt, for reasons that will be apparent in just a moment. Another study found it reduced sleep issues and improved sleep time, compared to a placebo (565). Ongoing research is exploring its role in reducing stress and anxiety. This supports its potential as a natural anxiolytic (567).

Common dosages of L-theanine are 100 to 200 mg per day. It is safe for most people, with a low risk of side effects. I will place a caveat on this statement though. For those with the COMT polymorphism V158M of the Met/Met (GG) genotype, l-theanine may be problematic. It raises dopamine levels, which are likely already too high. They have problems breaking it down when the gene is active (568).

I have also personally experienced issues with L-theanine because of mutations in my monoamine oxidase A (MAO-A) gene, which also breaks down dopamine, serotonin, and a couple of other neurotransmitters. Like people with COMT mutations, I tend to have trouble breaking down neurotransmitters. So, if I have L-theanine, I can put my brain into overload rather than calming it down.

Mutations in both of these genes are associated with ADHD, hence the warning about the study in the boys with ADHD

(569; 570). The study duration was six weeks, so it's unclear if it would have produced the same benefit long-term. If you have particular versions of the genes I've mentioned or diagnosed ADHD, it may promote wakefulness, not sleep. Approach with caution and, even if you find it works, try cycling it or only using it when absolutely necessary.

Saffron

Saffron has also been gaining attention for its potential benefits in improving sleep quality. Studies suggest that saffron may help with insomnia and overall sleep regulation due to its calming effects on the nervous system. Saffron contains active compounds like crocin and safranal, which influence neurotransmitters such as serotonin, known to promote relaxation and improve mood, which can, in turn, aid in falling and staying asleep (571).

Taking saffron 28-30mg of saffron as a supplement has been shown in some small studies to help reduce anxiety and improve overall sleep duration and quality, making it a natural option to consider for better rest (572). While more research is needed to solidify these claims, it's generally considered safe in moderate doses and has the added benefit of supporting mood stability and well-being as well.

But again, I'm going to recommend taking a cautious approach here and cycling it or only using it when necessary. This is especially true if you have COMT or MAO-A mutations such as those discussed with L-theanine. The reason for this is that it works a bit like selective serotonin reuptake inhibitors, preventing serotonins reuptake in the brain. This leaves more of it available to stimulate the neuroreceptor. Ultimately, there's a chance that this could lead to overstimulation of the serotonin system. It also seems to promote the release of dopamine and norepinephrine, which can also potentially result in overstimulation in some people.

I recommend to clients who use it that they cycle it for a period of time 1-2 months and use it as a sleep aid to help them reset their circadian rhythm. As such, I see it as beneficial for short-term use, but I suspect that long-term use may have unwanted side effects.

Prioritise Sleep

Until I began to get good sleep, I never knew how restorative it could be. These days, I acutely notice when something disturbs my sleep rhythm. The link between energy use, oxidative stress, and sleep shows how vital this restorative period is for our well-being. Sleep is not just a passive state. It is an active process. It is crucial for managing oxidative stress. It also ensures our body's resilience. In the end, it binds our health and vitality into a whole.

Activity

I'm sure you already know what I want you to do here. I want you to perform a subjective assessment on your sleep using the parameters I've outlined.

Go back through the chapter and give yourself a score from 1 to 5 for each parameter. 5 is the best score. If you give yourself a 5, then your work is done. But if you're anything less than a 4 or 5, you need to do some immediate work on the relevant area of your sleep. Use the tips I've provided here or do some googling. I guarantee improving your sleep will make a difference to how you feel.

Chapter Summary

- Sleep deprivation causes higher ROS levels and disrupts antioxidant production and repair mechanisms, leading to increased oxidative stress.
- Adequate sleep duration (7-9 hours) is essential for reducing oxidative stress and maintaining health.
- Sleep continuity is crucial; frequent awakenings disrupt sleep quality and can lead to various health issues.
- Strategies to improve sleep include optimising the sleep environment and managing factors such as alcohol consumption and nocturnal hypoglycaemia.
- Consistent sleep habits and adjustments tailored to individual needs are important for health and well-being.
- Cycling through light, deep, and REM sleep stages is crucial for maintaining healthy physiology and realising restorative sleep benefits.
- Non-REM sleep facilitates brain waste removal and growth hormone release, important for cellular repair.
- REM sleep plays a role in immune system regulation, reducing dysregulation and autoimmune symptoms.
- Waking up naturally after completing REM cycles can reduce grogginess and improve refreshment.

- Alcohol disrupts sleep cycles, particularly REM sleep, and should be consumed minimally and earlier in the evening.
- Exercise can extend REM sleep duration and improve sleep quality, as evidenced in studies involving rheumatoid arthritis.
- Sleep efficiency is the percentage of time spent asleep relative to time in bed, with high efficiency indicating better sleep quality.
- Consistent sleep and wake times regulate the circadian rhythm, hormone secretion, and improve sleep architecture.
- Regular sleep patterns support the release of growth hormone, essential for tissue repair and immune system modulation.
- Reducing blue light exposure, avoiding stimulating activities before bed, and engaging in relaxing activities like magnesium baths can aid sleep onset.
- Supplements like creatine, magnesium, saffron, and L-theanine can improve sleep quality and efficiency.
- Prioritising consistent and high-quality sleep is vital for managing oxidative stress and overall well-being.

Part 3 – Supporting Your Unique Biology

Where to From Here?

"A journey is a person in itself; no two are alike."

John Steinbeck

When I first got my diagnosis for Hashimoto's, I felt like my life was over. Having an autoimmune disease was liberating in a sense. I finally had answers about my health. But it also felt so final. I knew that life would go on, but I didn't have much hope that it would be better. From everything I'd read, once you had an autoimmune disease, you were stuck with it forever.

Then, I came across the paper about the epigenetic basis for autoimmune disease (573). I was bewildered. Everything else I'd read said that curing autoimmune disease was impossible. But I knew that if it was epigenetic, then there was a good chance that it could be reversed. That one paper was enough to give me a glimmer of hope and set me on this journey.

It also made me realise that I was going to have to go it alone. I couldn't afford to work with a holistic health practitioner then but had lost faith in doctors to treat chronic diseases. I did, however, find a great doctor who supported me with getting appropriate testing for a couple of years after my diagnosis.

But the actual healing bit? It was up to me to come up with a strategy and implement it.

You've already laid the groundwork to reverse your autoimmune disease in terms of lifestyle. Everything you've learnt and done so far has set you up for a much healthier future. What we're going to do now is take a look at how your genes might have predisposed you to autoimmune disease.

Note that there's no chapter summary here, because the chapter is structured a bit differently. Also, I think you must read the relevant parts in full.

I've left this bit until last for a couple of reasons, firstly, because I'm hoping that you've already put some lifestyle changes in place and started to notice a difference.

Secondly, because even though we're all genetically unique, these genetic differences only go so far. To be precise, there is a 0.1% between each of our genetic codes. That means that you and I are around 99.9% genetically the same (574).

What I've done so far is give you some general information that forms a solid foundation for improving your health and well-being. By adopting the changes already outlined, you should be well on your way towards better management or remission of your autoimmune disease. In fact, I put myself into full remission without what comes next, but I still had a few niggling problems afterwards. If I had done the steps outlined below sooner, I would have experienced greater health and vitality earlier.

Why are these nest steps so powerful? That 0.1% in genetic differences can still make a big difference in an acute situation. Especially when you have crucial differences in your methylation and detoxification genes.

We talked about these a little bit at the start of the book. But here's a quick recap.

Methylation genes control methylation. It is one of the three key processes that govern epigenetic expression. We know a lot about some mutations of the genes involved in methylation. They influence epigenetics, especially in the immune system. As I shared with you earlier, both hypo and hypermethylation are often issues that underpin autoimmune disease. This leads to dysregulated gene expression. In people with autoimmune disease, either can contribute to immune system overactivity.

As such, understanding these genes and supporting their proper function can help achieve optimal health and complete remission.

Detoxification genes do exactly what it sounds like they do. They help your body detoxify. They produce substances involved in neutralising and removing RS from your body. I'm sure you know by now exactly why this is important. Their job is to prevent oxidative stress. If they don't work well, you may have mitochondrial dysfunction, oxidative stress, and an overactive immune system.

What you're now going to learn about is the main pathways involved in the removal of RS from the body. Each of us has a unique genetic profile across these systems. Mutations in some of the genes involved can reduce the system's efficacy.

What this means is that you can have a genetic predisposition to an impairment in one of these systems. It may not be obvious though, until you find yourself in a situation where your detox systems are in overload. That's when the weakness will show via food or chemical sensitivity, neurological issues, or other symptoms you will soon learn are linked to problems in these systems.

Issues with methylation and detoxification often go hand-in-hand. There's a complex relationship between them. If there's a problem with one, then it's more than likely there will be a problem with the other.

But if you have problem mutations in your methylation or detox genes, I don't want you to panic. I can tell you, from having looked at many people's genetic profiles, that EVERYONE has problematic mutations in their genes. I'm yet to see a single perfect genetic profile.

It doesn't exist.

I also want to reassure you that you can have all kinds of problem mutations in methylation and detox genes yet still be perfectly healthy. Despite having pretty depressing methylation and detox panels, I've had periods of excellent health in my life. I also put myself into complete remission. If I can, so can you.

Everyone's situation is a little different. So, how you go about applying these next steps will be different. But the general strategies here will help. They address common issues with methylation and detoxification.

Below, you'll find an outline of the main systems involved in methylation and detoxification. I've added symptoms specific to each one to help you identify which are currently causing you the most issues. I've also included some supplements and foods to help get them working again. In some instances, I've noted foods or other substances that may also cause issues with these systems, so should be avoided if you think the relevant system is significantly impacting you. Following on from that, I've outlined how to do a detox to get these systems working again using the supplements and dietary strategies associated with each one.

What you should do now is go through each of these and make a note of which ones you think are causing you issues. At my worst, I might have ticked yes to all. But a few stood out. These are the ones that you should focus on - the ones that are causing you the most problems, while also being mindful of supporting the rest.

You may go through it with your doctor, a complementary medicine practitioner, or another health professional. Or it might be something you do all by yourself. Know if you need help, there are people out there who can support you. If you have questions, my social media, website, YouTube, or Medium and Substack articles may have the answers.

There are three major and three minor pathways that we're going to look at. The three major pathways are methylation, Phase I detoxification and Phase II detoxification. The minor pathways are glutathione, sulphuration, and n-acetylation, each of which feeds into Phase II detoxification. These are the main systems that your body uses to synthesise antioxidants and excrete toxins. There are others, but I've selected these ones because I think you'll get the most benefit from focusing on them.

Methylation takes place in all the cells in your body, whereas the majority of the detoxification processes take place in your liver. From there, most waste products are sent to the kidneys for filtering and excretion, though some are sent to the gallbladder and intestines for excretion in bile (575).

You can see how all of these processes are related in the diagram below.

Connections Between Detoxification Pathways

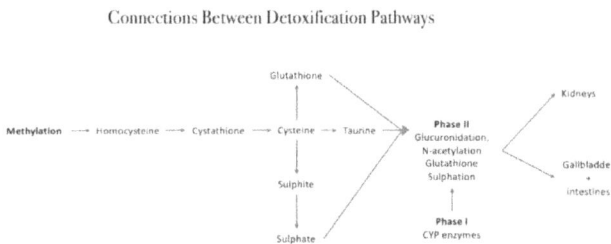

There are a number of general symptoms associated with issues in each of these pathways, as well as some that are specific to each pathway. Below I've listed the general symptoms that are common to all of these pathways.

- Fatigue and low energy
- Psychiatric disorders
- Cognitive issues (brain fog and trouble thinking)
- General digestive problems
- Hormonal imbalances (though you'll notice these are more

271

common/indicative in some than in others)
- Neurological symptoms
- Chronic pain.

I'm sure that you'll be nodding your head as you see this and saying yes, I have many (or all!) of those or have in the past. In addition, I've organised the symptoms more specifically to impairments in each pathway in the table below. It's worth noting that, while I haven't put it into the symptoms for all the other pathways, if the methylation pathway is impaired, it can have flow-on effects for all of these. The extent to which it does will depend on your specific genetic weaknesses, though.

Pathway	Symptoms
Methylation	Over or under-active immune system Cardiovascular problems, especially atherosclerosis Allergies Pregnancy complications, such as neural tube defects, preeclampsia, miscarriage (576; 577; 578; 579; 580)
CYP450/ Phase 1 detoxification	Unusual drug reactions or sensitivities Hormonal imbalances, including symptoms of hormonal disorders like PCOS and menopause-related symptoms (581)
Glucuronidation	Increased drug sensitivity Jaundice due to elevated levels of bilirubin, evident by yellowing of the skin and eyes Inability to metabolise dietary fats, may result in fatty liver Cardiomyopathy

	Hormonal imbalances due to buildup of sex hormones (582; 583)
Glutathione	Frequent infections
	Heavy metal toxicity
	Autoimmune diseases
	Poor regulation of blood sugar (584; 585; 586; 288)
Sulphation	Digestive issues accompanied by strong sulphur-smelling flatulence, especially after consumption of cruciferous vegetables, garlic and onions, animal protein, eggs, legumes, dairy, nightshades, and supplements that contain sulphur compounds
	Headaches and migraines
	Bad breath (halitosis)
	Body odour (noticeable sulphurous smell)
	Sensitivity to processed foods containing sulphites (indicator of an issue with SUOX) (587; 588; 589; 590; 591; 592)
N-Acetylation	Sensitivity to drugs (dizziness, nausea, organ damage)
	Trouble sleeping
	Histamine intolerance (593; 594)

Now that you've identified which of these pathways aren't working very well for you, you can read through the following section, focusing on the pathways that are most applicable to you. Remember, I've added in biomarkers so that you can do additional testing to check if you've correctly identified what's not working well for you. You can also compare your initial results against further testing over time as you make changes. I would recommend getting whichever of these biomarkers are the most relevant to you tested immediately so that you can make sure you're on the right track. From there, you can formulate a plan of what supplements you might need, foods or substances to avoid, and foods to include to get your detox pathways working again.

Personalising Your Detox Plan

Methylation Pathway

Methylation is crucial for DNA repair, detoxification, neurotransmitter synthesis, hormone regulation, and much more. We talked earlier about how impairments in methylation can lead to genes associated with immune function going haywire. This was back in the genetics section. But another thing associated with impaired methylation is impaired detoxification. The main reason is that methylation creates homocysteine, which we use to make cysteine. We talked about cysteine in the nutrition chapter during the discussion on protein: it's one of the three amino acids needed to generate glutathione. Cysteine also acts as the precursor to taurine and sulphite, which are used in Phase II and Sulphur detoxification pathways, respectively. So, methylation issues almost invariably go hand-in-hand with issues in all of these pathways (595; 596).

Most people will have some kind of genetic impairment in methylation. I have yet to see a single genetic panel that doesn't show a mutation that's potentially problematic for methylation. Several methylation genes can cause impairments, but the major one is MTHFR.

That said, there's a certain amount of redundancy built into the methylation cycle. This means if there's an issue somewhere, there tends to be another pathway that will mitigate that issue. Even if MTHFR isn't working well, other genes can pick up some of the slack, so long as they get the right substrates from your diet.

Below, we're going to have a look at some common biomarkers you can use to check your methylation status, plus foods and supplements to include to support methylation and what to avoid to support methylation.

Biomarkers to Check Methylation Status

- Homocysteine and/or S-adenosylhomocysteine (SAH) levels: Elevated homocysteine and/or SAH indicates methylation cycle dysfunction (597).
- Red blood cell folate (5-MTHF): Low levels suggest poor folate conversion and longer-term deficiency (598).
- Serum vitamin B12 (methylcobalamin): Low B12 levels indicate impaired methylation support (599).
- Other B vitamin deficiencies, as well as SAMe and choline deficiency (600).

Supplements to Support Methylation (601; 602)

- **Folate (Vitamin B9):** Folate is crucial for the methylation cycle as it provides methyl groups for the production of 5-methyltetrahydrofolate (5-MTHF), which donates a methyl group to homocysteine, converting it into methionine. This supports DNA methylation and gene expression regulation. In those with COMT (and some MAO-A) mutations, opt for folinic acid; for others, methyl folate should be suitable (603).
- **Methylcobalamin (Active B12):** Methylcobalamin acts as a cofactor for methionine synthase, an enzyme that converts homocysteine to methionine

by transferring methyl groups from 5-MTHF. This step is critical for maintaining proper methylation processes (604).

- **Betaine (trimethylglycine):** Betaine provides an alternative methylation pathway for homocysteine, helping to convert it into methionine when folate or B12 is deficient. It plays a key role in maintaining methylation balance in the body (605).
- **B-complex vitamins:** B vitamins, especially B2 (riboflavin), B6 (pyridoxine), and B3 (niacin), support the function of enzymes involved in methylation by providing cofactors for the remethylation of homocysteine and the conversion of methionine into SAMe (606).
- **SAMe (use with caution):** SAMe is the primary methyl donor in the body and is involved in over 100 methylation reactions, including DNA, RNA, and protein methylation, supporting many biological processes, including neurotransmitter synthesis and detoxification (607).

The best natural source of all of these (or, in the case of SAMe, its major substrate, methionine) is beef liver. I strongly recommend including it in your diet or taking it as a supplement as a long-term strategy rather than getting manufactured supplements if you have significant issues with methylation. It has so many other valuable nutrients in it as well and is easier on the body. I also deliberately haven't included quantities of each of these nutrients because the amount you should have is very individual and is based on your genetics and nutritional status. You need to do some reading on this and/or find a practitioner who can help you develop a tailored approach to methylation supplementation if you're not planning on consuming/supplementing with beef liver. This is especially true if you don't eat fish or animal-based products, as plant-based foods don't naturally contain B12.

Foods to Include to Support Methylation (148)

- Eggs
- Beef liver
- Muscle meats
- Leafy greens (organic, unwashed)
- Beetroot
- Shellfish
- Chickpeas.

Avoid the Following to Support Methylation

- Folic acid (the synthetic form of folate) in food or supplements.

Cytochrome P450 (Phase I) Detoxification Pathway

The Cytochrome P450 (CYP450) detoxification pathway is a crucial part of the body's ability to process and eliminate various substances, including drugs, toxins, and hormones. Think of it as a biochemical factory located primarily in the liver, where enzymes known as cytochrome P450 enzymes act as workers. These enzymes help modify harmful compounds. They do this by adding or changing specific chemical groups. This process turns fat-soluble substances into more water-soluble forms, which Phase II can then work on to make them ready to excrete through urine or bile.

When you take any medications, eat certain foods, or are exposed to toxins, the CYP450 enzymes spring into action. They convert these substances into less harmful compounds or even completely inactive forms (608). This detoxification process is vital for maintaining health, as it acts as the first stage of detoxification in the liver.

Next, we're going to go through biomarkers that can help you check if Phase I detoxification is working well for you, plus what you can add or remove to support it.

Biomarkers to Check Phase I Detoxification Status

- Liver function tests (ALT, AST): Elevated levels indicate impaired phase I detoxification (609).
- Drug sensitivity: Hypersensitivity to medications like SSRIs or beta-blockers can signal impaired CYP enzyme function (610).

Supplements to Support Phase I Detoxification

- **Milk thistle (silymarin):** Silymarin's role in Phase I detoxification can seem counterintuitive because it both inhibits and regulates cytochrome P450 enzymes, which are crucial for metabolising toxins in the liver. Preventing excessive activation that can lead to the formation of harmful reactive oxygen species (ROS). At the same time, it boosts antioxidant defences, particularly glutathione, to protect liver cells from oxidative damage during toxin metabolism (611; 612). This dual role helps maintain a balanced and less harmful detoxification process. 420mg/day supports liver detoxification and CYP function (613).

- **N-acetyl cysteine (NAC) + glycine:** NAC provides the body with cysteine, often the rate-limiting micronutrient in glutathione production. Glycine is a cofactor for the synthesis of glutathione, so taking these two in combination can enhance glutathione production. 100mg/kg body weight daily each helps balance phase I and phase II detoxification by boosting glutathione. Note that the 100mg is the *combined* dose of the two supplements together (i.e. 50mg +50mg/kg body weight) (614; 615).

Foods to Include to Support Phase I Detoxification (148)

- Cruciferous vegetables
- Citrus fruits
- Cantaloupe.

Avoid the Following to Support Phase I Detoxification

- Alcohol
- Caffeine
- Medications (do this safely, under guidance).

Phase II Detoxification

The Phase II detoxification pathway works closely with the Phase I pathway to help the body eliminate harmful substances, like drugs, toxins, and waste. In Phase I, CYP enzymes in the liver oxidise fat-soluble substances. This process often makes these substances less harmful or more water-soluble, but it can also produce more reactive metabolites that may need further processing.

Conjugation is a Phase II detoxification process where the body attaches a small molecule (such as glucuronic acid, sulphate, or glutathione) to toxins, making them more water-soluble and easier to excrete. In glucuronidation, glucuronic acid is added; in sulphation, sulphate is added; in glutathione conjugation, glutathione binds to toxins; and in N-acetylation, an acetyl group is added, all aiming to neutralise and eliminate harmful substances (575).

These pathways work together to detoxify a wide variety of compounds, including drugs, environmental toxins, and metabolic byproducts. I'll now go through each of them in more detail.

Glucuronidation Pathway

After the CYP450 enzymes modify unwanted substances, the glucuronidation pathway adds a sugar called glucuronic acid to them. This process makes the fat-soluble compounds more water-soluble. They can then be easily excreted through urine or bile. The enzymes involved in glucuronidation are uridine diphosphate-glucuronosyltransferases (UGTs). They act as a cleanup crew, neutralising and eliminating harmful substances from the body. Together, the CYP450 and glucuronidation pathways form a vital detoxification system that helps maintain overall health by ensuring that toxins and hormones (like estrogen) are efficiently processed and removed from the body, with glucuronidation being the most important of the Phase II processes as it accounts for around 40-60% of all conjugation activity (616).

Below, I've outlined the key biomarkers that indicate impaired glucuronidation, plus supplements and foods to include more of or avoid to support it.

Biomarkers to Check Glucuronidation Status
- Serum bilirubin: Elevated bilirubin levels suggest impaired UGT1A1 & UGT1A3 function (as seen in Gilbert's syndrome) (617).
- Hormone levels: Elevated oestrogen, especially oestradiol, may indicate impaired glucuronidation (618).
- Urinary hormone metabolites: Measure oestrogen and testosterone metabolites to assess clearance (619).
- Endometriosis, PCOS (620; 621) .

Supplements to Support Glucuronidation
- **Calcium D-glucarate:** Calcium d-glucarate supports glucuronidation by inhibiting the enzyme beta-glucuronidase, which reverses the glucuronidation process. By lowering beta-glucuronidase activity, calcium d-glucarate ensures that toxins bound to glucuronic acid are excreted efficiently rather than being reabsorbed into the body. This enhances the elimination of potentially harmful compounds, such as estrogen and carcinogens. 1000-1500mg/daily supports glucuronidation by inhibiting beta-glucuronidase,

an enzyme that breaks down glucuronic acid conjugates (622).

- **Berberine:** Berberine stimulates glucuronidation by enhancing the activity of UDP-glucuronosyltransferases (UGTs), the enzymes responsible for the glucuronidation of toxins and drugs. This helps to improve detoxification processes in the liver and facilitates the excretion of xenobiotics, including drugs, hormones, and other fat-soluble toxins. 1000-1500mg/daily helps break down estrogen metabolites, as well as being anti-parasitic and acting as an antioxidant (623).

- **Resveratrol:** Resveratrol also supports glucuronidation by modulating UGT enzyme activity, particularly UGT1A1. This aids in the conjugation of toxins, making them more water-soluble and allowing for their excretion via urine or bile. Additionally, resveratrol has been shown to increase the expression of enzymes involved in detoxification pathways, further supporting the glucuronidation process. 1000mg/daily increases UGT enzyme activity (624).

Berberine may not be the most suitable supplement for those with low estrogen. If you know you have symptoms of low estrogen, blood work reveals it's low, or you have a genetic mutation (as I do) that leads to fast estrogen metabolism, you have two options. The first is to avoid it and focus on other supplements instead. Or, take it with silymarin, to slow estrogen metabolism while allowing berberine to act on estrogen metabolites.

Foods to Include to Support Glucuronidation

- Cruciferous vegetables: Contain glucosinolates, which support glucuronidation (625).
- Oranges: Contains glucarate (622).

Avoid the Following to Support Glucuronidation

- Alcohol and acetaminophen: These substances inhibit UGT function, exacerbating detoxification issues (626).

Glutathione Detoxification Pathway

The glutathione detoxification pathway is a vital process in the body. It helps neutralise and eliminate harmful substances, such as toxins, heavy metals, and reactive oxygen species. Glutathione is a powerful antioxidant. It's made of three amino acids: cysteine, glutamine, and glycine, discussed in the nutrition chapter. Glutathione is in every cell, but especially the liver. It protects the body from oxidative stress and aids detoxification.

When harmful substances enter the body, glutathione binds to them, forming a compound that's easier to eliminate because they become water-soluble. This allows for their excretion through urine or bile. This process, called glutathione conjugation and which takes place in the liver, is vital for detoxifying many compounds, including drugs and toxins.

The body regenerates glutathione. This keeps levels high enough to handle daily toxins. Low glutathione levels can weaken detoxification and cause harmful substances to build up and increase health risks (627).

I've outlined biomarkers that can help you check how your glutathione pathway is functioning below, as well as what foods and supplements to include and things to avoid to support it.

Biomarkers to Check Glutathione Detoxification Status

- Glutathione levels (GSH): Low levels suggest impaired detox (628).
- Urinary organic acids: Elevated pyroglutamate (glutathione depletion marker) (629).
- Heavy metal tests: Elevated levels (e.g., mercury, lead) indicate reduced glutathione activity (630).

Supplements to Support Glutathione Detoxification

- **N-acetyl cysteine (NAC) + glycine:** NAC provides the body with cysteine, often the rate-limiting micronutrient in glutathione production. Glycine is a cofactor for the synthesis of glutathione, so taking these two in combination can enhance glutathione production. 100mg/kg body weight daily each boosts glutathione in those who need it. Note that the 100mg is the *combined* dose of the two supplements together (i.e. 50mg +50mg/kg body weight) (614; 615).
- **Alpha-lipoic acid:** ALA serves as both an antioxidant and a cofactor for mitochondrial enzymes. It supports the regeneration of glutathione

by recycling oxidised glutathione (GSSG) back into its reduced form (GSH). Through its interaction with the Nrf2/ARE signalling pathway, ALA enhances cellular defence mechanisms, including the upregulation of glutathione synthesis, offering protection against oxidative damage. 600mg/daily helps regenerate glutathione (631).

- **Selenomethionine or selenate:** Selenium is an essential cofactor for the enzyme glutathione peroxidase, which helps reduce hydrogen peroxide and lipid peroxides, using glutathione as a substrate. By providing selenium in the form of Selenomethionine or selenate, you ensure the proper function of glutathione peroxidase, thus maintaining antioxidant activity and preventing cellular damage caused by oxidative stress. 200mcg/daily enhances enzyme activity (632).

- **Liposomal or Intravenous Glutathione**: Both forms provide direct supplementation of reduced glutathione (GSH), which enhances the body's ability to neutralise free radicals and detoxify harmful substances. Liposomal glutathione has improved bioavailability compared to standard oral forms, while intravenous glutathione bypasses the digestive system entirely, delivering GSH directly into the bloodstream for immediate use by cells. 1000mg daily has been shown to increase glutathione levels (633).

Foods to Include to Support Glutathione Detoxification (148)

- Raw leafy greens (spinach, roquette)
- Beef liver
- Glutathione substrates (outlined in the nutrition chapter).

Avoid

- Alcohol
- Sugar
- Processes foods and chemicals
- Overconsumption of fatty fish with heavy metal contamination
- Caffeine.

Sulphation Pathway

The sulphation pathway is a key detoxification process. It helps eliminate harmful substances, like drugs, toxins, and hormones. This pathway adds a sulphate group (a molecule of sulphur and oxygen) to various compounds through conjugation. This makes them more water-soluble and easier for the body to excrete via urine. The liver mainly does this process using enzymes called sulfotransferases, which attach sulphate to unwanted molecules (634). Insufficient sulfotransferase activity due to taurine or zinc deficiency prevents effective sulphate processing, leading to sulphate accumulation.

However, issues in this pathway can arise earlier. A key step in the sulphation pathway is converting sulphites into sulphates. Sulphites are often produced during the breakdown of sulphur-containing compounds in the body. The conversion process is important because sulphites can be harmful in high amounts, whereas sulphates are safer and beneficial for detoxification. The enzyme sulphite oxidase (SUOX) converts sulphites into sulphates, allowing the sulphates to be used in the sulphation pathway (635). This conversion helps the body process and remove toxins, hormones, and waste. For people with mutations in the SUOX gene, getting enough molybdenum is extremely important.

Below, we're going to take a look at what you can do to check if your sulphation pathway is impaired, plus what supplements and foods you can either add more of or avoid to support it.

Biomarkers to Check Sulphation Detoxification Status

- Sulphate levels (blood/urine): Imbalance suggests impaired sulfation (636).
- Homocysteine levels: Elevated homocysteine can signal CBS or methylation issues (637).
- Urinary organic acids: High levels of sulphate and taurine can indicate sulphur imbalances (638).
- Zinc/copper deficiency: 900mcg/daily. Often associated with CBS polymorphisms AND the inability to detoxify sulphates (639; 640).

Supplements to Support Sulphation Detoxification

- **Molybdenum:** 45-500mcg/daily. Molybdenum is a cofactor for the enzyme sulphite oxidase (SUOX), which is critical in converting sulphites into sulphates. Without adequate molybdenum, sulphites can accumulate, leading to impaired detoxification and potentially toxic effects. By supporting SUOX activity, molybdenum ensures the proper metabolism of sulphur compounds, allowing sulphation processes to function effectively (641; 642).

- **Taurine:** 500-2000mg/daily. Taurine is a sulphur-containing amino acid that supports detoxification and cellular health, especially when sulphation is impaired. It helps in conjugating bile acids and may support the body's detoxification processes by enhancing the excretion of excess sulphur and other waste products, thus helping balance sulphur metabolism (643). Higher doses (1500mg) are useful in those with liver disease and hypertension (644).

- **Zinc:** Zinc is essential for the function of various enzymes involved in the sulphation pathway, including sulfotransferases, which are responsible for transferring sulphate groups to substrates such as hormones, drugs, and toxins. A zinc deficiency can reduce enzyme activity, impairing the sulphation pathway and leading to the inefficient breakdown of these compounds (645). It also reduces CBS activity in those with excess sulphites/sulphates and aids sulfotransferase activity. The recommended dose is 30-50mg/daily of zinc picolinate (639; 640).

- **Copper:** 900mcg/daily increases CBS activity in those with inadequate sulphates. Copper is essential as a cofactor for various enzymes, including CBS, which plays a role in the transsulphuration pathway that converts homocysteine into cystathionine and subsequently into cysteine. This pathway is critical for maintaining proper sulphur metabolism and supporting detoxification processes (639; 640).

Please don't supplement with copper or zinc unless you know you have a deficiency. They have a seesaw-like relationship in the body, where an excess of one can cause a deficiency in the other.

Foods to Include to Support Sulphation Detoxification (148)

- Chickpeas
- Beef liver
- Red meat
- Shellfish.

If you have sulphate excess, be a little cautious about adding too much sulphur-containing foods. Monitor yourself carefully until you find the right balance. Once you correct any micronutrient deficiencies, you will likely find that you can eat more of these foods.

Avoid the Following to Support Sulphation Detoxification

- Sugar and processed foods
- Alcohol
- Sulphur-containing foods (until the pathway is fully supported).

N-Acetylation Pathway

The N-acetylation pathway is a significant detoxification pathway in the body. This pathway modifies various xenobiotics (foreign compounds) and some natural substances through the production of enzymes by N-acetylation (NAT) genes. It adds an acetyl group, from acetyl-CoA, to the nitrogen atom of amines, which are the building blocks of some amino acids (646). One of the key compounds that it works on is the neurotransmitter serotonin. It helps your body turn serotonin into melatonin, which is important for sleep (647). Another amine to be aware of that it works on is histamine (648). There's a little bit of evidence that NAT2 genes play a role in histamine breakdown, so if you have histamine issues, there may be a problem with your N-acetylation pathway.

There are currently no tests publicly available to check this pathway's activity. Observe your symptoms and check your genetics. But, if you know you have issues with Phase II more generally, then chances are your N-acetylation will also be affected.

Below, I've outlined what foods and supplements can support this pathway, plus what to avoid to prevent its impairment.

Supplements to Support N-Acetylation Detoxification

- **Acetyl-L-Carnitine:** This compound not only aids in energy metabolism by transporting fatty acids into the mitochondria but also provides acetyl groups necessary for N-acetylation reactions.

Studies have shown that acetyl-L-carnitine can improve cognitive function and enhance mitochondrial health. A recommended dosage for cognitive support is 1,000 to 2,000 mg per day (649; 650).

- **Glycine**: As a non-essential amino acid, glycine acts as a substrate in N-acetylation and is critical for the synthesis of various compounds involved in detoxification, including glutathione. Glycine is known to support metabolic functions and has been studied for its potential benefits in sleep and cognitive function. A typical dosage is around 3,000 to 10,000 mg per day, often divided into doses (651; 652).

- **Choline**: This essential nutrient is crucial for the synthesis of phospholipids and acetylcholine, as well as providing methyl groups necessary for N-acetylation processes. Choline also supports liver function and lipid metabolism, making it beneficial for detoxification pathways. The recommended daily intake for choline is 425 mg for women and 550 mg for men (653).

- **N-acetyl cysteine (NAC) + glycine:** NAC provides the body with cysteine, often the rate-limiting micronutrient in glutathione production. Glycine is a cofactor for the synthesis of glutathione, so taking these two in combination can enhance glutathione production. 100mg/kg body weight daily, each boosts glutathione in those who need it. Note that the 100mg is the *combined* dose of the two supplements together (i.e. 50mg +50mg/kg body weight) (614; 615).

Foods to Include to Support N-Acetylation Detoxification (148)

- Avocadoes
- Nuts and seeds
- Red meat.

Avoid the Following to Support N-Acetylation Detoxification

- Processed meat
- Char grilled foods
- Synthetic chemicals, such as those outlined in section two during the discussion on environmental toxins.

How do you feel after reading about these detox pathways and seeing the diagram? Did anything jump out at you? Did you read one of these and say yes, that's me, I have most or all of those symptoms? If you have your genetic test handy, did your results match your symptoms?

Even if your symptoms don't match your genetics, don't discount them. It may be you're doing something right now to protect whatever problem genes you have. Find out what that is and keep doing it. Focus on the symptoms that you have right now.

I've given you suggested supplements for each of the pathways outlined. These can all be helpful if you have the associated symptoms. But I want you to note that these aren't long-term solutions. Most of them should only be used in the short term (with a couple of exceptions, which I'll discuss).

You MUST get the basic lifestyle factors already discussed in this book right to be healthy. This includes eating the foods recommended to support each of these pathways (unless you can't for some medical reason). You'll still be hanging by a thread if all you do is take some of the supplements mentioned in this section.

It's also crucial you read the next section before going out and buying any supplements. Why? Because there's an order to doing things so that you get the best outcome with the least harm.

Preparing for a Detox

It may be necessary to undertake a detox protocol for a short period to help your body catch up. Here, you eliminate foods and substances that cause you issues. At the same time, you add supplements and foods that boost your detox pathways. If multiple detox pathways are presenting major issues for you, you need to address them ALL.

Make sure that if you do this, you've addressed any micro (or macro) nutrient deficiencies first. Your body needs to be well-nourished to undertake any kind of detoxification.

Copper is the exception. It's important to pathogen growth, so if you have mould or bacterial imbalances, you want to wait until you're rid of them before you take a copper supplement (654).

The one caveat that I would mention is this: *leave the methylation cycle alone initially.*

Yes, you read that right. Leave the methylation cycle alone until after you've got the rest of the cycle working better. Why? Because the last thing you want to do is end up with a backlog of additional homocysteine that your body can't use. This is just going to make things worse.

If you can't work with a good practitioner to identify deficiencies, the e-book called *How to Interpret Your Blood Test Results,* which I mentioned during the nutrition chapter, teaches you how to do this. You'll find a link to it on my website. I've designed it to easily identify most major micronutrient deficiencies. You can do this using general tests that your doctor can order without raising their eyebrows. Also, labs set their ranges based on a link to disease, not optimal health and detoxification. You need a diagnosable condition, like liver disease, for their ranges to show anything. My experience has taught me issues can arise in any of these systems without a full-blown medical crisis.

If you lack key nutrients to make antioxidants, detox will be useless. It will make you feel worse than you did at the start, and, in all honesty, it won't work very well. Many people tell me their detox experiences were ineffective or unpleasant.

This is the reason why.

Their body wasn't prepared for it.

After identifying problematic detox systems and addressing nutrient deficiencies (3-6 weeks), you have two options. Find a natural or holistic therapist. They should be experienced in detoxification. I highly recommend this. It's good to have someone to call on if you have questions or if something goes wrong, especially if you have the added complication of a parasite issue.

The other option is to do it yourself. I've outlined how to do this below, but I want to stress to you that this isn't medical advice. If you go it alone, please do extra research. Monitor yourself carefully. Get help from a practitioner immediately if you have problems.

Detoxifying

Barring methylation substrates, get the supplements needed to do a detox. You don't necessarily need all those I've listed with each detox pathway, I've just included a few to give you some options. This is where working with a naturopath or another holistic practitioner may be useful, as they may be able to devise or recommend a clean formulation that works well for you and is readily accessible based on your specific symptoms and any deficiencies.

You can also find formulations with herbs and compounds that support most of these pathways off the shelf in chemists or online. If you're buying something like this, though, I would recommend looking for something that comes in a capsule so that you can avoid getting any binders or fillers. Some people can be quite sensitive to these, so if that's you, be extra selective about what you buy.

You may also find that certain companies use different formulations with different herbs than what I've recommended here. This is fine, but I would recommend doing some reading or asking a holistic practitioner to ensure you're getting something that's powerful enough to work without overwhelming your detox systems AND targets the systems that you know are problematic for you.

Mould and Histamine Issues
If you have a mould and/or histamine issue, then I would recommend dealing with this first or concurrently. Some of the supplements listed above will help with mould, but it's such a tricky issue that I would recommend working with someone who can walk you through the process of getting rid of it concurrent with doing a detox. Alternatively, I have a mould protocol on my website, which is also suitable for those with histamine issues, which you can use in conjunction with what we're about to go over.

Heavy Metal Toxicity

If you have a heavy metal toxicity issue, it's important to do this at the same time as well. The best product that I can recommend for this is modified citrus pectin (MCP). It's a soluble fibre derived from the peel and pulp of citrus fruits. Regular pectin molecules are large and are not easily absorbed by the body, but MCP is specially modified to have a lower molecular weight, making it more bioavailable and allowing it to enter the bloodstream. It's thought to work by binding to certain receptors in the body, especially one called galectin-3. High levels of galectin-3 are linked to inflammation, fibrosis, and certain cancers, so it's quite a powerful anti-inflammatory. It also chelates to heavy metals, helping to remove them from the body.

There's not a huge amount of research on MCP, though one small study has shown that it increases the rate of heavy metal excretion from the body without depleting essential minerals and also has protective effects against cancer (655; 656). This makes it extremely safe. It's also much gentler than some other products used for heavy metal detoxification. And there is plenty of anecdotal practitioner data on its efficacy.

How much should you take? The study cited above showed that 15g/day, broken down into 5g doses across the day, was effective. Some anecdotal evidence suggests that a higher dose can help remove heavy metals faster if you want to complete a detox quickly (in just a few weeks), but the problem with this is that then your detox pathways have more to excrete all at once. If you have an autoimmune disease, they're probably already dealing with a lot. I recommend 15-20g/day across a longer period (1-3 months) so that you're not overburdening your system. It will bind to some of the nutrients in your food, so make sure to have it at least half an hour post-meal or a few hours before food.

Additionally, it may well be worth taking some activated charcoal concurrently. Activated charcoal is a form of charcoal processed to have small, low-volume pores that increase its surface area, allowing it to adsorb toxins and chemicals in the body when ingested or applied topically. It can act as a binding agent, helping you remove heavy metals once MCP has chelated them. A typical dose is 500-1000mg 1-3 times per day. Make sure not to have it with food, though, as it can end up binding to the nutrients you eat (657). Instead, as with the MCO, have it between meals but also separate to the MCP.

Liver Support

Another compound I recommend you take that doesn't directly work on any of these pathways but supports liver function more generally is inositol, otherwise known as vitamin B8. You can get it directly from fresh (uncooked and unfrozen) fruit, or as a supplement.

It does many different things in the body, including indirect contributions to methylation and Phase I detoxification. It comes in different forms – the more common form is Myo-inositol, but some people can't metabolise this into its active form. If you take it and don't notice an effect, D-chiro-inositol may work better for you. 2-4g daily is the recommended dose (658; 659).

Support Bowel Function

If you're frequently constipated or your bowel movements are irregular, magnesium may also be helpful. The reason why is that it can relax the intestine and draw water into the bowel, which promotes bowel movements. Try 200-400mg/day of magnesium citrate. Even if you don't have issues with your bowel movements, it's advisable to eat plenty of foods high in magnesium during a detox for the same reason. Leafy greens, nuts and seeds, legumes, and dark chocolate are all good sources (660). Just be careful of too much magnesium if your kidneys aren't working well.

The other thing that's worth considering if you have issues with bowel movements is eating foods with natural probiotics. Think kefir, live yoghurt, sauerkraut, and kimchi. They can bolster your microbiome and also aid with improving bowel movements (661). Note I'm not advocating that you go out and get probiotics in pill form. There's a real art to supplementing with the kind of probiotics you buy, and sometimes, supplementing with the wrong type can cause more problems than it solves, especially if you have histamine intolerance. Stick with probiotics in food form unless you're working with a practitioner who can help you choose the right strains for your symptoms and/or stool analysis. However, if you have histamine issues, stay away from fermented foods and focus on the rest.

You must get your bowel working before or during a detox so that the toxins in your body will have somewhere to *go*. There's no point freeing them up, but then they just sit in your body and cause other problems.

How to Support Yourself During a Detox
Avoid any foods you're sensitive to so you don't add more stress to your system. Also, eat more of the recommended foods.

Sometimes, you might have two conflicting systems. A food that helps one is causing problems in another. Avoid these foods completely, even if it means that your diet is a little more limited. But please be careful not to miss out on any of the macro or micronutrients your body needs to function. You'll achieve better results if your body is fully nourished.

You also need to do the following things during a detox to support yourself.

1. **Drink plenty of water**, more than you normally would. Drink up to double your recommended amount. This will help with the removal of any RS that your detox frees up and

support your kidneys. If you don't get enough water, RS may linger in your body. This can cause more side effects and prolong the detox experience. Make sure to get enough salt to support the extra fluid intake.

2. **Balance your electrolytes.** If electrolytes are imbalanced (which you'll see through your hair mineral analysis), it can be difficult for your cells to expel RS and keep them out for removal by your detoxification organs. Imbalanced electrolytes can also predispose you to more mast cell reactions (more info on this in my MCAS course online).

3. **Eat plenty of fibre**. Fibre can bind to RS and help excrete them from the body.

4. **Get your body moving**, but don't push too hard. We discussed the need for movement. It boosts your antioxidants and lymphatic system. So, you know why it's important. In saying that, don't push yourself too hard beyond your normal threshold, as this can add overload to your detox systems at a time when they're already busy.

5. **Prioritise sleep and rest**. The last thing you want to do during a detox is impair detoxification further by adding extra stress to your detox systems. As we've discussed, sleep is incredibly important for the removal of RS from your body. So, is there any other time

when your metabolism is less active? It means your RS production will go down. This lets your antioxidants and detox systems catch up.

6. **Use the emotion regulation technique** discussed in the nervous system chapter or some other type of breathwork or meditation to help you regulate emotions and stay grounded. The process of detoxification can add stress to your body, so you need to fully support yourself emotionally.

Beginning the Detox

Take any supplements in the morning and at lunch, at least initially, so that you can monitor if you have any adverse reactions. I would also recommend having them with food so that they're not acting on an empty stomach. In addition, if you're on medication, check in with your doctor or specialist and do some reading to make sure none of these will interfere with your medications.

Rather than taking everything all at once, I suggest you incorporate each new supplement slowly. Each time you add a new one in, wait 2-3 days before adding in the next one. This will allow you to monitor how you feel with each new addition. If anything feels terrible straight away, decrease the dose and build your way up slowly. If there's something that just doesn't work for you, leave it out.

This is especially true if you have severe mast cell activation symptoms, which can lead to allergic reactions that become anaphylactic. Be EXTREMELY careful if this is you. If you have lupus or any other autoimmune disease that directly affects liver, kidney, gallbladder, or intestinal function, I advise taking things slowly there as well so that you're not overloading an already struggling system.

At the end of the day, always pay attention to how you feel.

Unfortunately, even though you've done some prep work, you might have a bit of a rough time with the detox. Any of the symptoms associated with the detox pathways outlined previously may increase a little during the detox period, at least initially. But if you experience any severe symptoms, you're likely pushing yourself too hard. Trust me, I know this from personal experience. Decrease the amount of everything you're having to a point where it's tolerable, and be prepared instead for a longer but gentler detox period.

If any adverse symptoms last longer than a couple of weeks, STOP. Wait for a month or two before trying again. During the waiting period, stick with any dietary changes you've made for the detox so long as you can meet your nutritional needs. Continue taking any micronutrient supplements and keep on being careful and gentle with yourself.

The amount of time that you need to spend doing a detox is very individual. Generally, the worse your symptoms, the longer your detox will need to go because you probably have more accumulated RS. Anywhere from a month and up to two or three months may be necessary. Give yourself at least two months, but longer if you feel that things still aren't quite where you want them. Keep up with the supplements for at least a week after you feel like you're ready to stop.

Post-Detoxification

After you stop the detox, you want to carefully reintroduce any foods you've been avoiding. Throughout a couple of weeks, reintroduce them one by one. Just add one more in every 3-4 days and monitor how you feel. If you have some kind of an adverse reaction, back it off, give yourself a couple more days, and then try again with a smaller dose.

This is the point at which you can think about kicking your methylation into gear if it's not working all that well. Now that your detoxification systems are working properly, you shouldn't end up with a homocysteine accumulation, which is a good sign of issues with methylation. But you might also find that you don't need to do anything other than focus on getting the right foods in your diet – supplementation may very well not be necessary. This is because, even though methylation will almost certainly have been sub-optimal while you were sick, now that you're well, you'll be making fewer demands on the system.

Before charging in with supplements to help with methylation, I advise getting some general bloodwork done and looking over it with a holistic practitioner or comparing them against my guide. This will show your overall progress, including how well your methylation and detox pathways are functioning. Hopefully, you'll be feeling better by this point, but it's well worth checking that things are running smoothly.

However, if you feel that things are still a little suboptimal or bloodwork shows that any of your B vitamins might be low, you can support methylation with a grass-fed liver supplement. If, for some reason, you're not keen on this or can't get it, try some B vitamins as supplements, just be a little cautious and make sure to introduce any new supplements slowly. These, plus creatine for general health and molybdenum for those with sulphite intolerance, are the only supplements mentioned in this worth considering long-term due to the demands of modern life. In saying that, I want to reiterate once more that supplementation is no replacement for diet. Chances are, if you're not getting enough B vitamins from your diet, you won't be getting enough of other things as well, so try and support yourself as much as possible with food.

By the time the detox is over, I hope that you'll be feeling a lot more invigorated and energised. It can take a little while for some of your biomarkers to stabilise and for tissue to heal. This is especially true if you've had hormonal issues. But, if you stick with the principles outlined in section 2 of the book beyond any detox period, you should see constant improvements in your health.

Now would be a good time to go back and take a look at your results from the questionnaires and exercises you did earlier, at the end of some of the chapters. You might find it interesting to do some of them again, such as those at the end of the chapters on your environment, nutrition, and sleep. You could also make note of any improvements in sleep and movement practices. But perhaps the most interesting of all will be to retake the quizzes on oxidative stress and immune system function. Also, have another look at your heart rate variability, as outlined at the end of the nervous system chapter.

How have things changed for you? How does it feel to see those changes?

Is there anything that hasn't worked well for you? Make a note and learn from it. And if you'd like to reach out and let me know, please do. I'd love to hear your feedback so I can continually make subsequent versions of this book better. I have a contact form on my website that you can use.

Last thing: *celebrate your wins.*

You deserve to because these conditions can be awful to deal with. Make sure that you congratulate and give yourself the credit you deserve for making progress. Healing yourself takes a lot of courage, especially when you may have faced resistance from family, friends, and even your medical team. You should be proud of yourself for making it this far.

Conclusion

"You will always fail. But inside of doing that, you will advance and advance and advance... I watched a fight once and a guy lost 14 rounds in a row and knocked the guy out in the 15th round. That takes heart."

Walter Mosley

If you've made it this far, I thank you and applaud you. You've gotten through a lot of information. By now, you have a much better understanding of the epigenetic basis for autoimmune disease, how your immune system creates autoimmune disease and the role of oxidative stress and the antioxidant defence system. You know how your nervous system plays a part in autoimmune disease onset and maintenance. You also understand how important your emotional health, diet, environmental health, movement, and sleep are to managing and reversing your condition. You have some specific guidelines and recommendations around what you can do to improve your health through addressing issues in each of these areas. And you know why methylation and detoxification genes are so important. They often hold the key to autoimmune disease. You know how to check if they're an issue for you, and what you need to do to address them.

Hopefully, you're feeling confident by now that you can do this. You can manage your autoimmune symptoms or possibly even put it into remission. You have a list of actionable steps that you can take over time, crossing them off slowly as you bring them into your life. You're well-equipped to make the changes needed to take charge of your health.

But here's the problem. Things might not go quite right. Something that's out of control might knock the stuffing out of you and push you back into old habits. The numbers on your blood tests might get better then stall. They may even get worse if something really big pushes you over the edge.

I want you to know that setbacks and pitfalls are inevitable. They happen. To everyone. Even me.

For the first two years after I found out that I had an autoimmune disease, life was fairly breezy. I had a couple of blips like when I had a really bad allergic reaction to incense my flatmate gave me. That had me in bed for three days, barely able to breathe, let alone think or move. I accidentally ate gluten a couple of times and spent a few days recovering. I had a stressful period where I had to decide if I wanted to finish my PhD, eventually deciding against it. But on the whole, my recovery was progressing pretty well.

Then two years in, I had a major setback. I moved to the other side of the country to be with my partner. While this meant I was in a loving and supportive relationship, there were several drawbacks to the move. I was now within about an hour of where I had been living when I first got sick and developed CPTSD. This was very traumatic for me. At the same time, I changed the structure of my business, plus we started to go into the post-COVID economic downturn. I also let go of my exercise routine and changed my diet slightly. For all of these reasons, I went through a terrible time and could see some of my CPTSD symptoms flaring up again. My physical health seemed to be slipping too. The accumulation of all of these stressors was sending me backwards.

After about six months of this, I realised that I really needed to change something, otherwise I might lose all the ground I'd gained over the last few years. I got myself back into a routine with exercise and readjusted my diet. I started changing my business structure back to how it was before and got a part-time job to help pay bills while the economy sucked. Finally, I started my Masters of Counselling and got qualified in nutrition and complementary medicine. All of this took about six months to put into action and then longer to execute some of it. I didn't do it in a day, but I did it because I chose life and health and love.

The crazy thing is, I learnt so much through that little setback. I learnt my priorities and what I thought I could do with my career to help people had changed. I discovered that I was much better than I previously thought at running my own business. It also made me realise the importance of my diet and exercise routine.

I spent time in places and around people who previously terrified me and... nothing happened. I lived to tell the tale. Better yet, I embarked on a whole new set of adventures, like the certifications I've since done to become a complementary medicine practitioner. I set new directions for my business and ran a marathon! I made awesome new friends that I'm sure I'll have for life. And I wrote this book!

And as you already know, I still managed to get myself into remission.

My point is, you're more than likely going to experience some setbacks on your healing journey. They will batter and bruise you; they might even knock you down for a while. But don't lose sight of your end goal.

I promise you, if you keep on getting back up, and looking for new ways to win, you will succeed. Your life, that life which is uniquely yours, is the most precious and rare thing you will ever have within your grasp. Whatever it takes, however you need to nourish and care for yourself to live it and live it well – it will be worth it.

Remember, you've committed a day in your future life to paper. Your entire being knows where you want to go. Your task now is to give yourself what you need to get there.

Acknowledgements

There are so many people I need to thank here!

A huge thank you to Pascal Gambardella, who read through and helped edit every single page of this book. Without your help, it would have been a lot harder to read and probably been too technical for most people to understand. I sincerely appreciate the time and effort you put into reading and providing me with feedback.

Thanks also to my writing mentor, Neeramitra Reddy. In a short space of time, you've taught me the power of my own experience, how to use my voice, and pushed me to be that little bit more vulnerable in my writing. I know that I've reached and helped more people because of you.

Thank you to those who so generously shared your experiences with me. Living with an autoimmune condition is isolating and traumatic. Thank you for trusting me with your stories.

I also need to thank my clients, who have taught me so much in such a short space of time. Every new person who comes to me presents a unique challenge and provides a valuable learning experience along the way.

I would also like to thank my family and friends, who have listened to me talking about autoimmune diseases and chronic health issues for years now! Somehow, they don't get sick of me and continually want to hang out and catch up. Thank you for your ongoing support.

I would also like to thank my former PhD supervisors, Kirsten Martinus, Marit Kragt, and Natasha Paulie. They haven't had a direct hand in this book, and my PhD was on a different topic, but working with them reinvigorated my love of research and connecting the dots. They also gave me focus and goals at a time when I was struggling to find my place in the world.

I also need to thank my friend Jamie Doughney. You saw a light in me when even I was blind to it. I'm not sure I would have made it through a very dark time without the ray of hope that you gave me.

And last but not least. Thank you to Joe, my partner, who has so patiently sat and listened to me, talking about my discoveries and insights, my progress, and my sticking points in writing this book. I'm so grateful to you every day for being the person that you are.

About the Author

Lou Chalmer is a former environmental scientist and winemaker turned psychosomatic counsellor and nutrition and genetics consultant based in Victoria, Australia.

After overcoming her own autoimmune issues and battle with mental health, she realised that everything she'd learnt through her journey was too valuable not to share it. This prompted her career change, which included further study to increase her knowledge and to gain qualifications to work directly with clients.

A big proponent of the notion of self-organising complex systems, she believes that the body has the inherent ability to heal itself from many wounds and incursions. This includes those caused by autoimmune attacks on the self. Her approach is about giving the body what it needs to reorganise itself and return to homeostasis.

In her spare time, she loves to cook, read, keep fit, and spend time in nature.

Bibliography

1. *The Increasing Prevalence of Autoimmunity and Autoimmune Diseases: An Urgent Call to Action for Improved Understanding, Diagnosis, Treatment and Prevention.* **Miller, F.M.** 2023, Curr Opin Immunol., Vol. 80.

2. *Environmental triggers and autoimmunity.* **Vojdani, A. and Pollard, K.M., Campbell, A.W.** s.l. : Autoimmune Dis. , 2014.

3. **ASCIA.** Autoimmune Diseases - Fast Facts. *ASCIA.* [Online] June 2023. https://www.allergy.org.au/patients/fast-facts/autoimmune-diseases.

4. —. Autoimmune Diseases - Fast Facts. *Australasian Society of Clinical Immunology & Allergy.* [Online] June 2023. https://www.allergy.org.au/patients/fast-facts/autoimmune-diseases.

5. *Toxicities of immunosuppressive treatment of autoimmune neurologic diseases.* **Lallana, E.C. and Fadul, C.E.** 2011, Curr Neuropharmacol., pp. 468-77.

6. *Therapy Side Effects in Systemic Lupus Erythematosus.* **Popa, R., et al.** 3, 2018, Curr Health Sci J. , Vol. 44, pp. 316-321.

7. *Steroids are a risk factor for Kaposi's sarcoma-immune reconstitution inflammatory syndrome and mortality in HIV infection.* **Fernández-Sánchez, M., et al.** 6, s.l. : AIDS, 2016, Vol. 30. 909-14.

8. *"I was never like that": Australian findings on the psychological and psychiatric sequelae of corticosteroids in haematology treatments.* **McGrath, P., Patton, M.A. and James, S.** s.l. : Supportive Care in Cancer, 2008, Vol. 17. 339–347.

9. *Standards of Medical Care in Diabetes—2022 Abridged for Primary Care Providers.* **American Diabetes Association.** 1, s.l. : Clinical Diabetes, 2022, Vol. 40. 10–38.

10. *Subclinical disease activity in systemic lupus erythematosus: immunoinflammatory markers do not normalize in clinical remission.* **Wais, T., et al.** 10, s.l. : J Rheumatol., 2003, Vol. 30. 2133-9.

11. *Towards personalized medicine for patients with autoimmune diseases: Opportunities and challenges.* **Tavakolpour, S.** s.l. : Immunology Letters, 2017, Vol. 190. 130-138.

12. **American Autoimmune Association.** Path to a Rare Disease Diagnoses. [Online] October 2021. https://autoimmune.org/resource-center/autoimmune-summit/2021-autoimmune-summit/path-to-rare-disease-diagnoses/.

13. *The complexity of autoimmune disease: Diagnostic and therapeutic considerations.* **Benson, K. and Haines, J.** 1, 2006, Journal of Autoimmunity, Vol. 26, pp. 21-33.

14. *Diagnosis and management of autoimmune disease.* **Krupp, L. B. and Elkins, M.** 2, 2008, Current Opinion in Rheumatology, Vol. 20, pp. 137-143.

15. *Understanding patient experiences in chronic illness management: A systematic review.* **Morris, A. and Lankford, J.** 7-8, 2015, Journal of Clinical Nursing, Vol. 24, pp. 1013-1022.

16. **Coatsworth, N.** Don't protest too loudly, doctors - we do have a Medicare crisis. *The Sydney Morning Herald.* [Online] 19th October 2022. https://www.smh.com.au/national/don-t-protest-too-loudly-doctors-we-do-have-a-medicare-crisis-20221018-p5bqtb.html.

17. **Afrin, L.** *Never Bet Against Occam.* s.l. : Self-published, 2016.

18. *Is there time for management of patients with chronic diseases in primary care?* **Østbye, T., et al.** 2, s.l. : Ann Fam Med., 2005, Vol. 3. 209-14.

19. *An Assessment of Clinically Useful Measures of the Consequences of Treatment.* **Laupacis, A., Sackett, D.L.**

and **Roberts, R.S.** 26, 1988, The New England Journal of Medicine, Vol. 318.

20. *American College of Rheumatology. Preliminary definition of improvement in rheumatoid arthritis.* **Felson, D.T., et al.** 6, 1995, Arthritis Rheum., Vol. 38, pp. 727-35.

21. *Randomised double-blind placebo-controlled study of interferon β-1a in relapsing/remitting multiple sclerosis.* **Ebers, G.C.** 9139, 1998, The Lancet, Vol. 352, pp. 1498-1504.

22. *Mechanisms of neuronal dysfunction and degeneration in multiple sclerosis.* **Dutta, R. and Trapp, B.D.** 1, s.l. : Prog Neurobiol., 2011, Vol. 93.

23. *Number Needed to Treat Network Meta-Analysis to Compare Biologic Drugs for Moderate-to-Severe Psoriasis.* **Leonardi, C.L., et al.** 5, 2022, Adv Ther., Vol. 39, pp. 2256-2269.

24. *nfection risk associated with anti-TNF-α agents: a review.* **Murdaca, G., et al.** 4, s.l. : Expert Opin Drug Saf. , 2015, Vol. 14.

25. *Chronic inflammation in the etiology of disease across the life span.* **Furman, D., et al.** s.l. : Nat Med, 2019, Vol. 25, pp. 1822-1832.

26. *Immunogenicity of Biologics in Chronic Inflammatory Diseases: A Systematic Review.* **Strand, V., et al.** 4, s.l. : BioDrugs, 2017, Vol. 31.

27. *Comparing Biologic Cost Per Treated Patient Across Indications Among Adult US Managed Care Patients: A Retrospective Cohort Study.* **Gu, T., et al.** 4, s.l. : Drugs Real World Outcomes, 2016, Vol. 3.

28. **Department of Health and Aged Care.** *Therapeutic Goods Administration - Financial and non-financial performance.* s.l. : Australian Government, 2021.

29. **Brown, S.** Most Dietary Guideline Advisors Have Ties to Food and Pharma Industries, Study Finds. *Very Well Health.* [Online] 22nd March 2022. https://www.verywellhealth.com/dietary-guidelines-committee-conflicts-of-interest-

5223556#:~:text=Key%20Takeaways&text=A%20new%2
0report%20found%20that,available%20on%20the%20Diet
ary%20Guidelines..

30. **Sims, S.** Women are Not Small Men: a paradigm shift in the science of nutrition. *TED x Talks : Youtube.* [Online] 24th September 2019. https://www.youtube.com/watch?v=e5LYGzKUPlE.

31. *Cardiovascular disease in women: A statement for healthcare professionals from the American Heart Association.* **Wenger, N. K.** 8, 2009, Circulation, Vol. 119, pp. 1211-1222.

32. *Gender and health care: The effects of patient gender on medical decision-making.* **Miller, A. G., Hogg, M. A. and Marquardt, M. J.** 6, 2001, Health Psychology, Vol. 20, pp. 494-501.

33. *Gender differences in autoimmune disease prevalence: An overview.* **Saddi, R., Bae, S. and Kelley, J.** 12, 2019, Autoimmunity Reviews, Vol. 18, p. Autoimmunity Reviews.

34. *The role of women in health care.* **Becker, M. H. and Murphy, L. B.** 6, 2000, Journal of Women's Health, Vol. 9, pp. 565-572.

35. *Gender, sex, and health: What are the connections—and why does it matter?* **Krieger, N.** 4, 2003, International Journal of Epidemiology, Vol. 32, pp. 652-653.

36. **Stairs, L.** The dismissal and disbelief of women living with autoimmune diseases significantly impacts time to diagnosis and proper treatment. *American Autoimmune Association.* [Online] 8th March 2022. https://autoimmune.org/its-all-in-your-head-recognizing-the-plight-of-women-living-with-autoimmune-diseases-on-international-womens-day/.

37. **Ministers Department of Health and Aged Care.** 2 out of 3 women experience discrimination in healthcare. *Australian Government.* [Online] 14th March 2024. https://www.health.gov.au/ministers/the-hon-ged-kearney-

mp/media/2-out-of-3-women-experience-discrimination-in-healthcare-0.

38. **ACA.** *Scope of practice for registered counsellors.* 2020.

39. *Trauma in the Mind and Pain in the Body: Mind-Body Interactions in Psychogenic Pain.* **Sima, A. and Hosier, S.** 1, s.l. : Human Architecture : Journal of the Sociology of Self - Knowledge, 2011, Vol. 9. 111-131.

40. **Pert, C.B.** *Molecules of Emotion: The Science Behind Mind-Body Medicine.* s.l. : Scribner, 1997.

41. **Means, C. and Means, C.** *Good Energy: The Surprising Connection Between Metabolism and Limitless Health.* s.l. : Avery Publishing Group, 2024.

42. **Rankin, L.** *Mind Over Medicine: Scientific Proof That You Can Heal Yourself.* s.l. : Hay House, 2020.

43. *Homeostatic Control of the Thyroid-Pituitary Axis: Perspectives for Diagnosis and Treatment.* **Hoermann, R., et al.** 177, s.l. : Front Endocrinol (Lausanne), 2015, Vol. 6.

44. *Serum TSH, T(4), and thyroid antibodies in the United States population (1988 to 1994): National Health and Nutrition Examination Survey (NHANES III).* **Hollowell, J.G., et al.** 2, s.l. : J Clin Endocrinol Metab., 2002, Vol. 87, pp. 489-99.

45. **Department of Health.** Thyroid - Hashimoto's disease. *Better Health Channel.* [Online] Victoria State Government, 6th December 2011. https://www.betterhealth.vic.gov.au/health/conditionsandtreatments/thyroid-hashimotos-disease.

46. *A spontaneous remission of Hashimoto's thyroiditis.* **Trimeche, O., et al.** s.l. : Endocrine Abstracts, 2024, Vol. 99.

47. **Carnivore Diet.** Tracey Reversed Her Hashimoto's On A Carnivore Diet. [Online] 5th May 2022. https://carnivore.diet/tracey-reversed-her-hashimotos-on-a-carnivore-diet/.

48. **Gawain, S.** *Creative Visualisation.* s.l. : New World Library, 1978.

49. **Huberman Lab.** Dr. Martha Beck: Access Your Best Self With Mind-Body Practices, Belief Testing & Imagination. *YouTube.* [Online] 5th August 2024. https://www.google.com/url?sa=t&source=web&rct=j&opi =89978449&url=https://www.youtube.com/watch%3Fv%3 DnOgypsWKjm4&ved=2ahUKEwi7r7vly_- HAxWuRmwGHeucPA0QwqsBegQICxAG&usg=AOvVa w08yxAQMc_vzJikaAzZaNef.

50. **Tim Ferriss Show.** How to Design a Life — Debbie Millman . *Tim Ferriss.* [Online] 12th January 2017. https://tim.blog/2017/01/12/how-to-design-a-life-debbie- millman/.

51. **Alberts, B., et al.** *Molecular Biology of the Cell (4th ed.).* s.l. : Garland Science, 2002.

52. **Lodish, H., et al.** *Molecular Cell Biology (4th ed.).* s.l. : W. H. Freeman, 2000.

53. **Nelson, D. L., & Cox, M. M.** *Lehninger Principles of Biochemistry (4th ed.).* s.l. : W. H. Freeman, 2005.

54. **NIH.** Understanding Human Genetic Variation. [Online] National Library of Medicine, 2007. [Cited: 28 May 2024.] https://www.ncbi.nlm.nih.gov/books/NBK20363/.

55. *Transducing bioelectric signals into epigenetic pathways during tadpole tail regeneration.* **Tseng, A.S. and Levin, M.** 10, 2012, Anat Rec (Hoboken), Vol. 295, pp. 1541-51.

56. *Endogenous bioelectrical networks store non-genetic patterning information during development and regeneration.* **Levin, M.** 11, 2014, The Journal of Physiology, Vol. 592, pp. 2295-2305.

57. *Two Forms of Electrical Transmission Between Neurons.* **Faber, D.S. and Pereda, A.E.** 427, 2018, Front Mol Neurosci., Vol. 11.

58. *Epigenetics: A Landscape Takes Shape.* **Goldberg, A.D., Allis, C.D. and Bernstein, E.** 4, 2007, Cell, Vol. 128, pp. 635-638.

59. *DNA methylation patterns and epigenetic memory.* **Bird, A.** 1, 2022, Genes & Development, Vol. 16, pp. 6-21.

60. *Translating the Histone Code.* **Jenuwein, T. and Allis, C. D.** 5532, 2001, Science, Vol. 293, pp. 1074–1080.

61. *Genome regulation by long noncoding RNAs.* **Rinn, J. L. and Chang, H. Y.** 1, 2012, Annual Review of Biochemistry, Vol. 81, pp. 145–166.

62. *Bioelectric mechanisms in regeneration: Unique aspects and future perspectives.* **Levin, M.** 5, 2009, Semin Cell Dev Biol., Vol. 20, pp. 543-56.

63. *Mendelian disorders of the epigenetic machinery: postnatal malleability and therapeutic prospects.* **Fahrner, J.A. and Bjornsson, H.T,.** R2, 2019, Human Molecular Genetics, Vol. 28, pp. R254–R264.

64. *Understanding Critical Periods in Development.* **Smith, J.** 3, 2020, Journal of Developmental Biology, Vol. 8, p. 18.

65. *Bioelectric controls of cell proliferation: Ion channels, membrane voltage and the cell cycle.* **Blackiston, D.J., McLaughlin, KA. and Levin, M.** 21, 2011, Cell Cycle, Vol. 8, pp. 3519-3528.

66. *Cracking the bioelectric code: Probing endogenous ionic controls of pattern formation.* **Tseng, A. S. and Levin, M.** 1, 2013, Communicative & Integrative Biology, Vol. 6.

67. **Lipton, B. H.** *The Biology of Belief.* s.l. : Hay House, 2008.

68. *Genetic and epigenetic fine mapping of causal autoimmune disease variants.* **Farh, K.K.H. and et al.** s.l. : Nature, 2014, Vol. 518. 337-343.

69. *The emerging role of epigenetics in human autoimmune disorders.* **Mazzone, R. Zwergel, C., et al.** 2019, Clinical Epigenetics, Vol. 11.

70. *Updated assessment of the prevalence, spectrum and case definition of autoimmune disease.* **Hayter, S. M. and Cook, M. C.** 10, 2012, Autoimmunity Reviews, Vol. 11, pp. 754-765.

71. *Autoimmune diseases.* **Davidson, A. and Diamond, B.** 5, 2001, New England Journal of Medicine, Vol. 345, pp. 340-350.

72. **Johns Hopkins Medicine: Pathology.** Disease Development: How do Autoimmune Diseases Unfold? [Online] 2024. [Cited: 18 May 2024.] https://pathology.jhu.edu/autoimmune/development#:~:text=Results%20have%20shown%20that%20there,considered%20polygenic%20(multifactorial)%20diseases..

73. **Rose, N. R. and Mackay, I. R.** *The Autoimmune Diseases (4th ed.).* s.l. : Academic Press, 2004.

74. *HLA association with autoimmune disease: a failure to protect?* **Zanelli, E., Breedveld, F.C. and de Vries, R.R.P.** 10, s.l. : Rheumatology, 2000, Vol. 39, pp. 1060–1066.

75. —.**Zanelli, E., Breedveld, F.C. and de Vries, R.R.P.** 10, 2000, Rheumatology, Vol. 39, pp. 1060–1066.

76. *A genetic perspective on coeliac disease.* **Trynka, G., Wijmenga, C. and van Heel, D.A.** 11, 2010, Trends Mol Med., Vol. 16, pp. 537-50.

77. *The shared epitope hypothesis. An approach to understanding the molecular genetics of susceptibility to rheumatoid arthritis.* **Gregersen, P.K., Silver, J. and Winchester, R.J.** 11, 1987, Arthritis Rheum., Vol. 30, pp. 1205-13.

78. *Robust associations of four new chromosome regions from genome-wide analyses of type 1 diabetes.* **Todd, J.A. and et al.** 7, 2007, Nat Genet., Vol. 39, pp. 857-64.

79. *Recent insights in the epidemiology of autoimmune diseases: Improved prevalence estimates and understanding of clustering of diseases.* **Cooper, G. S., Bynum, M. L. and Somers, E. C.** 3-4, 2009, Journal of Autoimmunity, Vol. 33, pp. 197-207.

80. *Genome sequencing in clinical practice: Applications, challenges, and opportunities.* **Ramos, E. M., & Shedlock, K.** 3, 2019, Dialogues in Clinical Neuroscience, Vol. 21, pp. 239-252.

81. *Bisulfite genomic sequencing: systematic investigation of critical experimental parameters.* **Grunau, C., Clark, S.J. and Rosenthal, A.** 13, 2001, Nucleic Acids Res., Vol. 29, pp. E65-5.

82. *Association between Genetic Polymorphisms in Methylenetetrahydrofolate Reductase and Risk of Autoimmune Diseases: A Systematic Review and Meta-Analysis.* **Lu, M., et al.** 2022, Disease Markers.

83. *Epigenome-wide association data implicate DNA methylation as an intermediary of genetic risk in rheumatoid arthritis.* **Liu, Y., et al.** 2013, Nat Biotechnol, Vol. 31, pp. 142–147.

84. *Global DNA methylation, DNMT1, and MBD2 in patients with systemic lupus erythematosus.* **Liu, C., et al.** 2011, Lupus, Vol. 20, pp. 131–136.

85. *Towards an understanding of the role of DNA methylation in rheumatoid arthritis: therapeutic and diagnostic implications.* **Cribbs, A., Feldmann, M. and Oppermann, U.** 5, 2015, Therapeutic Advances in Musculoskeletal Disease, Vol. 7, pp. 206–219.

86. *DNA methylation signatures of autoimmune diseases in human B lymphocytes.* **Zouali, M.** 2021, Clinical Immunology, Vol. 222.

87. *MTHFR mutations in female patients with autoimmune thyroiditis.* **Bulgar, A., et al.** 2011, Endocrine Abstracts, Vol. 26, p. 210.

88. *A candidate genetic risk factor for vascular disease: a common mutation in methylenetetrahydrofolate reductase.* **Frosst, P., et al.** 1, 1995, Nature Genetics, Vol. 10, pp. 111-113.

89. *A second common mutation in the methylenetetrahydrofolate reductase gene: an additional risk factor for neural-tube defects?* **van der Put, N. M. J., et al.** 5, 1998, American Journal of Human Genetics, Vol. 62, pp. 1044-1051.

90. *Functional analysis of genetic variation in catechol-O-methyltransferase (COMT): effects on mRNA, protein, and enzyme activity in postmortem human brain.* **Chen, J., et al.** 5, 2004, American Journal of Human Genetics, Vol. 75, pp. 807-821.

91. *The role of DNA methylation in mammalian epigenetics.* **Jones, P. A. and Takai, D.** 5532, 2001, Science, Vol. 293, pp. 1068-1070.

92. *Mutations in the RNA polymerase II transcription machinery: insights into the pathogenesis of disease.* **Wen, H. and Manley, J. L.** 5, 2012, Molecular cell, Vol. 10, pp. 295-305.

93. *Mortality in randomized trials of antioxidant supplements for primary and secondary prevention: systematic review and meta-analysis.* **Bjelakovic, G., et al.** 8, 2007, Jama, Vol. 297, pp. 842-857.

94. *Role of mitochondria in non-alcoholic fatty liver disease.* **Pessayre, D.** Suppl 1, 2007, Journal of Gastroenterology and Hepatology, Vol. 22, pp. S20-S27.

95. *Association of hyperhomocysteinemia with genetic variants in key enzymes of homocysteine metabolism and methotrexate toxicity in rheumatoid arthritis patients.* **Chaabane, S., et al.** s.l. : Inflamm. Res., 2018, Vol. 67.

96. *Association of COMT Val158Met Polymorphism with Fibromyalgia in Khartoum State, Sudan.* **Mamoun Abdelmageid, S., et al.** s.l. : Pain Res Manag., 2023. 37305098.

97. *Homocysteine imbalance: a pathological metabolic marker.* **Schalinske, K.L. and Smazal, A.L.** 6, s.l. : Adv Nutr., 2012, Vol. 3, pp. 755-62.

98. *Combination Effect of GSTM1, GSTT1 and GSTP1 Polymorphisms and Risk of Systemic Lupus Erythematosus.* **Salimi S, Nakhaee, A., et al.** 6, s.l. : Iran J Public Health. , 2015, Vol. 44.

99. *Single-nucleotide polymorphisms (SNPs) of antioxidant enzymes SOD2 and GSTP1 genes and SLE risk and severity in an Egyptian pediatric population.* **Abd El Azeem, R.A., et al.** s.l. : Clinical Biochemistry, 2021, Vol. 88, pp. 37-42.

100. *Impact of NQO1 dysregulation in CNS disorders.* **Yuhan, L., Khaleghi Ghadiri, M. and Gorji, A.** s.l. : Journal of Translational Medicine, 2024, Vol. 22.

101. *The impact of CYP2C9 and VKORC1 genetic polymorphism and patient characteristics upon warfarin dose requirements: proposal for a new dosing regimen.* **Sconce, E. A., et al.** 7, 2005, Blood, Vol. 106, pp. 2329-2333.

102. *The role of genetic polymorphisms in the pharmacokinetics and pharmacodynamics of tacrolimus.* **Hesselink, D. A., et al.** 10, 2003, Clinical Pharmacokinetics, Vol. 52, pp. 825-857.

103. *Interaction between folate and aging in disease.* **Choi, S. W. and Friso, S.** 5, 2005, Clinics in Geriatric Medicine, Vol. 21, pp. 621-639.

104. *Role of metabolic H2O2 generation: redox signaling and oxidative stress.* **Sies, H.** 13, 2014, J Biol Chem., Vol. 289, pp. 8735-41.

105. *Hormesis and Oxidative Distress: Pathophysiology of Reactive Oxygen Species and the Open Question of Antioxidant Modulation and Supplementation.* **Nitti, M. and et al.** . 8, 2022, Antioxidants, Vol. 11.

106. *Oxidants, oxidative stress and the biology of ageing.* **Finkel, T. and Holbrook, N.J.** 6809, 2000, Nature, Vol. 408, pp. 239-47.

107. *Reactive Oxygen Species in the Immune System.* **Yang, Y., et al.** 2013, International Reviews of Immunology, Vol. 3, pp. 249-270.

108. *Hydrogen peroxide as a central redox signaling molecule in physiological oxidative stress: Oxidative eustress.* **Sies, H.** 2017, Redox Biol., Vol. 11, pp. 613-619.

109. *Reactive oxygen species (ROS) homeostasis and redox regulation in cellular signaling.* **Ray, P. D., Huang, B. W. and Tsuji, Y.** 5, 2012, Cell Signal, Vol. 24, pp. 981-990.

110. *Oxidative stress and ion channel modulation: A review on the mechanisms of altered electrophysiological properties in cardiac hypertrophy and heart failure.* **Chaudhary, P., Sinha, K. and Banerjee, D.** 2017, Frontiers in Cardiovascular Medicine, Vol. 4, p. 19.

111. *ROS-mediated modulation of ion channels.* **Wang, Q., Tiwari, P. and Bradley, R.** 2019, Cell Calcium, Vol. 84, pp. 102-110.

112. *Membrane changes under oxidative stress: the impact of oxidized lipids.* **Itri, R., et al.** 1, 2014, Biophys Rev., Vol. 6, pp. 47-61.

113. *Transcriptional deregulation by oxidative stress.* **Sen, S. and Ghosh, S.** 6, 2013, Antioxidants & Redox Signaling, Vol. 18, pp. 618-636.

114. *Role of S-adenosylmethionine in liver health and injury.* **Mato, J. M., Corrales, F. J. and Lu, S. C.** 1, 2002, Advances in Nutrition, Vol. 35, pp. 1-9.

115. *Epigenetics: A new bridge between nutrition and health.* **Choi, S. W., Friso, S. and Choi, J. W.** 1, 2011, Advances in Nutrition, Vol. 2, pp. 8-16.

116. *Crosstalk of reactive oxygen species and NF-κB signaling.* **Morgan, M. J. and Liu, Z. G.** 1, 2011, Cell Research, Vol. 21, pp. 103-115.

117. **Berg, J. M., Tymoczko, J. L. and Stryer, L.** *Biochemistry (7th ed.).* s.l. : W.H. Freeman, 2012.

118. *How mitochondria produce reactive oxygen species.* **Murphy, M. P.** 1, 2009, Biochemical Journal, Vol. 417, pp. 1-13.

119. *The control region of mitochondrial DNA shows an unusual CpG and non-CpG methylation pattern.* **Bellizzi, D., et al.** 5, 2012, DNA Research, Vol. 19, pp. 537-547.

120. *Mitochondria as sensors and regulators of calcium signalling.* **Rizzuto, R., et al.** 9, 2012, Nature Reviews Molecular Cell Biology, Vol. 13, pp. 566-578.

121. *Metabolism and role of glutamate in mammalian brain.* **Erecinska, M. and Silver, I. A.** 4, 1990, Progress in Neurobiology, Vol. 35, pp. 245-296.

122. *Oxidative stress: Free radical production in neural degeneration.* **Götz, M. E., et al.** 1, 2018, Pharmacology & Therapeutics, Vol. 63, pp. 37–122.

123. *Mitochondrial formation of reactive oxygen species.* **Turrens, J. F.** 2, 2003, Journal of Physiology, Vol. 552, pp. 335–344.

124. *Mitochondrial outer-membrane protein FUNDC1 mediates hypoxia-induced mitophagy in mammalian cells.* **Liu, L., et al.** 2, 2013, Nature Cell Biology, Vol. 14, pp. 177–185.

125. *Mitochondrial pathology: Stress signals from the energy factory.* **Raimundo, N.** 5, 2014, Trends in Molecular Medicine, Vol. 20, pp. 282-292.

126. *Mitochondrial pathology: stress signals from the energy factory.* **Raimundo, N.** 5, s.l. : Trends Mol Med., 2014, Vol. 20.

127. *Mitochondria in health, disease, and aging.* **Harrington, J.S., et al.** 4, 2023, Physiol Rev., Vol. 103, pp. 2349-2422.

128. **McDowell, H. and Volk, A.A.** Infant Mortality. [book auth.] S.L. Hart and D.F. (eds) Bjorklund. *Evolutionary Perspectives on Infancy.* s.l. : Springer, 2022, pp. 83–103\.

129. **Hurtado, A.M.** *Ache Life History: The Ecology and Demography of a Foraging People.* s.l. : Routledge, 1996.

130. *Reproductive trade-offs in extant hunter-gatherers suggest adaptive mechanism for the Neolithic expansion.* **Page, A.E., et al.** 17, 2016, Proc Natl Acad Sci U S A, Vol. 113, pp. 4694-9.

131. *Life history theory and the immune system: Steps toward a human ecological immunology.* **McDade, D.W.** S37, 2003, American Journal of Biological Anthropology, Vol. 122, pp. 100-125.

132. *Old Meets New: The Interaction Between Innate and Adaptive Immunity.* **Clark, R. and Kupper, T.** 4, 2005, Journal of Investigative Dermatology, Vol. 125, pp. 629-637.

133. *Oxidative stress: A concept in redox biology and medicine.* **Sies, H.** 11, 2017, Redox Biology, pp. 613-619.

134. *Adaptive homeostasis.* **Davies, K.J.A.** 2016, Molecular Aspects of Medicine, Vol. 49, pp. 1-7.

135. *Redox regulation of mitochondrial biogenesis.* **Piantadosi, C.A. and Suliam, H.B.** 11, 2012, Free Radical Biology and Medicine, Vol. 53, pp. 2043-2053.

136. *Meta-analytic evidence for increased low-grade systemic inflammation and oxidative stress in hypothyroid patients. Can levothyroxine replacement therapy mitigate the burden?* **Tellechea, M.L.** 2021, Endocrine, Vol. 72, pp. 62–71.

137. *Cytokines in autoimmunity: role in induction, regulation, and treatment.* **Moudgil, K. D. and Choubey, D.** 1, 2018, Journal of Interferon & Cytokine Research, Vol. 38, pp. 1-2.

138. **Kumar, V., et al.** *Robbins Basic Pathology E-Book.* s.l. : Elsevier Health Sciences, 2018.

139. *Autoimmune Disorders–A Review of Current and Future Drugs and Therapies.* **Bhattacharyya, S., Kumar, A., Lal, M., & Verma, D.** 2, 2018, Austin Therapeutics, Vol. 5, p. 1057.

140. *The development of allergic inflammation.* **Galli, S.J., Tsai, M. and Piliponsky, A.M.** 7203, 2008, Nature, Vol. 454, pp. 445-54.

141. *Mast cells.* **Metcalfe, D.D., Baram, D. and Mekori, Y.A.** 4, 1995, Physiol Rev., Vol. 77, pp. 1033-79.

142. **Janeway, C. A., et al.** *Immunobiology: The Immune System in Health and Disease (5th ed.).* s.l. : Garland Ed., 2001.

143. *Innate immune recognition: mechanisms and pathways.* **Medzhitov, R. and Janeway, C. A.** 1, 2000, Immunological Reviews, Vol. 173, pp. 89-97.

144. *Diagnosis, presentation, and management of mast cell activation syndrome.* **Afrin, L. B.** 4, 2020, Current Allergy and Asthma Reports, Vol. 20.

145. *Doctor, I Think I Am Suffering from MCAS: Differential Diagnosis and Separating Facts from Fiction.* **Valent, P. and Akin, C.** 4, 2019, The Journal of Allergy and Clinical Immunology: In Practice, Vol. 7, pp. 1109-1114.

146. *Mast cell activation syndromes: definition and classification.* **Valent, P.** 4, s.l. : Allergy, 2013, Vol. 68, pp. 417-24.

147. **National Institutes of Health.** Dietary Supplement Fact Sheets. [Online] 2021. https://ods.od.nih.gov/factsheets/list-all/.

148. **NIH.** Nutrient Recommendations and Databases. [Online] https://ods.od.nih.gov/HealthInformation/nutrientrecommen dations.aspx.

149. *Quercetin is more effective than cromolyn in blocking human mast cell cytokine release and inhibits contact dermatitis and photosensitivity in humans.* **Weng, Z., et al.** 3, s.l. : PLoS One., 2012, Vol. 7.

150. *Quercetin as a Dietary Supplementary Flavonoid Alleviates the Oxidative Stress Induced by Lead Toxicity in Male Wistar Rats.* **Al-Zharani, M., et al.** 8, s.l. : Nutrients, 2023, Vol. 15.

151. *Anti-allergic effect of vitamin C through inhibiting degranulation and regulating TH1/TH2 cell polarization.* **Li, Q., et al.** 10, Journal of the Science of Food and Agriculture : s.n., 2024, Vol. 104, pp. 5955-5963.

152. *The novel flavone tetramethoxyluteolin is a potent inhibitor of human mast cells.* **Weng, Z., et al.** 4, s.l. : J Allergy Clin Immunol., 2015, Vol. 135, pp. 1044-1052.

153. *In vitro anti-inflammatory effects of curcumin on mast cell-mediated allergic responses via inhibiting FcεRI protein expression and protein kinase C delta translocation.* **Kong, Z.L., et al.** 1, s.l. : Cytotechnology, 2020, Vol. 72, pp. 81-95.

154. *Quercetin increased bioavailability and decreased methylation of green tea polyphenols in vitro and in vivo.* **Wang, P., Heber, D. and Henning, S.M.** 6, s.l. : Food Funct., 2012, Vol. 3, pp. 635-42.

155. *Interactions between the microbiota and the immune system.* **Hooper, L.V., Littman, D.R. and Macpherson, A.J.** 6086, 2012, Science, Vol. 336, pp. 1268-73.

156. *Genetic and epigenetic influences on the loss of tolerance in autoimmunity.* **Zhang, P. and Lu, Q.** 2018, Cellular & Molecular Immunology, Vol. 15, pp. 575–585.

157. *Autoimmune effector memory T cells: the bad and the good.* **Devarajan, P. and Chen, Z.** 2013, Immunologic Research, Vol. 57, pp. 12–22.

158. *Stressors, stress, and neuroendocrine integration of the adaptive response: The 1997 Hans Selye Memorial Lecture.* **Chrousos, G.P.** 1998, Ann N Y Acad Sci., Vol. 851, pp. 311-35.

159. *Cardiac coherence: A new, noninvasive measure of autonomic nervous system order.* **Tiller, W.A., McCraty, R. and Atkinson, M.** 1, 1996, Alternative Therapies in Health and Medicine, Vol. 2, pp. 52-65.

160. **Margulis, L. and Sagan, D.** *Microcosmos.* s.l. : University of California Press, 1997.

161. *Controller-regulator model of the central nervous system.* **Ito, M.** 2, 2002, J Integr Neurosci. , Vol. 1, pp. 129-43.

162. **Nicholls, J. G., et al.** *From Neuron to Brain.* s.l. : Sinauer Associates, 2012.

163. *Neurotransmitter release: The last millisecond in the life of a synaptic vesicle.* **Südhof, T. C.** 3, 2013, Neuron, Vol. 80, pp. 675-690.

164. *The central autonomic nervous system: conscious visceral perception and autonomic pattern generation.* **Saper, C.B.** 2002, Annu Rev Neurosci., Vol. 25, pp. 433-69.

165. **Purves, D., et al.** *Neuroscience.* s.l. : Oxford University Press, 2018. Vol. 6th ed.

166. *Psychoneuroimmunology: The science of the mind-body connection.* **Ader, R.** 2, 2007, Current Directions in Psychological Science, Vol. 16, pp. 79-83.

167. **Damasio, A.** *Feeling and Knowing: Making Minds Conscious.* s.l. : Robinson, 2023.

168. **Waxenbaum, J.A., Reddy, V. and Vacarello, M.** Statpearls: Anatomy, Autonomic Nervous System. [Online]

NIH, 24 July 2023. [Cited: 18 May 2024.]
https://www.ncbi.nlm.nih.gov/books/NBK539845/.

169. *Sympathetic and parasympathetic indicators of heart rate control at altitude studied by spectral analysis.* **Hughson, R.L., et al.** 6, 1994, J Appl Physiol , Vol. 77, pp. 2537-42.

170. **Goldstein, D.S.** *The Autonomic Nervous System in Health and Disease.* s.l. : CRC Press, 2000.

171. *Measures of sympathetic and parasympathetic autonomic outflow from heartbeat dynamics.* **Valenza, G., et al.** Journal of Applied Physiology : s.n., 2018, Journal of Applied Physiology, Vol. 125, pp. 19-39.

172. **Barton Furness, J.** *The Enteric Nervous System.* s.l. : Hohn Wiley & Sons, 2008.

173. *Methods of assessing vagus nerve activity and reflexes.* **Chapleau, M.W. and Sabharwal, R.** 2010, Heart Failure Reviews, Vol. 16, pp. 109-127.

174. *The polyvagal perspective.* **Porges, S.W.** 2, 2007, Biol Psychol., Vol. 74, pp. 116-43.

175. **Janig, W.** *Integrative Action of the Autonomic Nervous System: Neurobiology of Homeostasis.* Cambridge : Campbridge University Press, 2006.

176. *Emotion regulation: Affective, cognitive, and social consequences.* **Gross, J. J.** 3, 2002, Psychophysiology, Vol. 39, pp. 281-291.

177. **Dana, D.A.** *The Polyvagal Theory in Therapy: Engaging the Rhythm of Regulation.* s.l. : Norton Agency Titles, 2018.

178. *Homeostasis and Self-Tolerance in the Immune System: Turning Lymphocytes off.* **Van Parijs, L. and Abbas, A.K.** 5361, 1998, Science, Vol. 280, pp. 243-248.

179. *A body–brain circuit that regulates body inflammatory responses.* **Jin, H., et al.** 2024, Nature, Vols. https://www.nature.com/articles/s41586-024-07469-y.

180. *Sympathetic neural-immune interactions regulate hematopoiesis, thermoregulation and inflammation in*

mammals. **Madden, KS..** 2017, Dev Comp Immunol., Vol. 66, pp. 92-97.

181. *Beyond heart rate variability: Vagal regulation of allostatic systems.* **Thayer, J. F. and Sternberg, E.** 1, 2006, Annals of the New York Academy of Sciences, Vol. 1088, pp. 361-372.

182. *Physiology and neurobiology of stress and adaptation: Central role of the brain.* **McEwen, B. S.** 3, 2007, Physiological Reviews, Vol. 87, pp. 873-904.

183. **McCraty, R. and Childre, D.** Clinical applications of the coherence research. *Heartmath.* [Online] https://www.heartmath.org/.

184. *Psychosocial interventions and immune function: A review.* **Schwartz, M. S. and et al.** 2, 2010, Health Psychology Review, Vol. 4, pp. 155-175.

185. *The inflammatory reflex.* **Tracey, K.J.** 6917, 2002, Nature, Vol. 420, pp. 853-9.

186. *From inflammation to sickness and depression: when the immune system subjugates the brain.* **Dantzer, R., et al.** 1, 2008, Nat Rev Neurosci., Vol. 9, pp. 46-56.

187. *Mitochondrial Dysfunction: At the Core of Psychiatric Disorders?* **Andreazza, A.C. and Nierenberg, A.A.** 9, 2018, Biol Psychiatry, Vol. 83, pp. 718-719.

188. *Immune dysregulation.* **Long, A., Kleiner, A. and Looney, R.J.** 1, 2023, Journal of Allergy and Clinical Immunology, Vol. 51, pp. 70-80.

189. *A healthy heart is not a metronome: an integrative review of the heart's anatomy and heart rate variability.* **Shaffer, F., McCraty, R. and Zerr, C.L.** 2014, Frontiers in Pscyhology, Vol. 5.

190. *Heart Rate Variability: Measurement and Clinical Utility.* **Kleiger, R.E., Stein, P.K. and Bigger Jr., J.T.** 1, 2005, Annals of Noninvasive Electrocardiology, Vol. 10, pp. 88-101.

191. *Cardiac coherence, self-regulation, autonomic stability, and psychosocial well-being.* **McCraty, R. and Zayas, M.A.** 2014, Frontiers in Psychology, Vol. 5.

192. *Is heart rate a convenient tool to monitor over-reaching? A systematic review of the literature.* **Bosquet, L., et al.** 9, 2009, British Journal of Sports Medicine, Vol. 42, pp. 709-714.

193. **Harari, Y.N.** *Sapiens.* s.l. : Harper, 2015.

194. *Regional differences in synaptogenesis in human cerebral cortex.* **Huttenlocher, P.R. and Dabholkar, A.S.** 2, s.l. : J Comp Neurol., 1997, Vol. 387, pp. 167-78.

195. *Temporal and spatial dynamics of brain structure changes during extensive learning.* **Draganski, B., et al.** 23, 2006, The Journal of Neuroscience, Vol. 26, pp. 6314-6317.

196. *Co-morbidity and systemic inflammation as drivers of cognitive decline: new experimental models adopting a broader paradigm in dementia research.* **Cunningham, C. and Hennessy, E.** 1, s.l. : Alzheimers Res Ther. , 2015, Vol. 7.

197. *Trauma-Related Dissociation and the Dissociative Disorders:: Neglected Symptoms with Severe Public Health Consequences.* **Boyer, S.M., Caplan, J.E. and Edwards, L.K.** 2, 2022, Dela J Public Health., Vol. 8, pp. 78-84.

198. **Levine, P.** *Waking the Tiger: Healing Trauma: The Innate Capacity to Transform Overwhelming Experiences .* s.l. : North Atlantic, 2011.

199. *Effects of childhood trauma on working memory in affective and non-affective psychotic disorders.* **Quidé, Y., et al.** 2017, Brain Imaging and Behavior, Vol. 11, pp. 722–735.

200. *Retrospective Reports of Childhood Trauma in Adults With ADHD.* **Rucklidge, J. J., et al.** 4, 2006, Journal of Attention Disorders, Vol. 9, pp. 631-641.

201. *Borderline personality disorder and childhood trauma: Evidence for a causal relationship.* **Ball, J.S. and Links, P.S.** 2009, Curr Psychiatry Rep, Vol. 11, pp. 63–68.

202. **Van der Kolk, B.** *The Body Keeps the Score.* s.l. : Penguin Books, 2014.

203. **Mate, G.** *Scattered Minds: The Origins and Healing of Attention Deficit Disorder.* s.l. : Vermilion Books, 2019.

204. *Heart and Brain Interaction of Psychiatric Illness: A Review Focused on Heart Rate Variability, Cognitive Function, and Quantitative Electroencephalography.* **Jung, W., Jang, K.I. and Lee, S.H.** 4, 2019, Clin Psychopharmacol Neurosci., Vol. 17, pp. 459-474.

205. *Inflammation-related biomarkers in major psychiatric disorders: a cross-disorder assessment of reproducibility and specificity in 43 meta-analyses.* **Yuan, N., et al.** 1, 2019, Transl Psychiatry, Vol. 9, p. 233.

206. *Relationship of childhood abuse and household dysfunction to many of the leading causes of death in adults.* **Felitti, V.J., et al.** 4, 1998, Am J Prev Med, Vol. 14, pp. 245-58.

207. *Cumulative childhood stress and autoimmune diseases in adults.* **Dube, S.R., et al.** 2, 2009, Psychosom Med., Vol. 71, pp. 243-50.

208. *Posttraumatic stress disorder and risk of selected autoimmune diseases among US military personnel.* **Bookwalter, D.B., et al.** 1, 2020, BMC Psychiatry, Vol. 20, p. 23.

209. *Association of Stress-Related Disorders With Subsequent Autoimmune Disease.* **Song, H., et al.** 23, 2018, JAMA, Vol. 319, pp. 2388–2400.

210. *Sleep is for Foregetting.* **Poe, G.R.** 3, 2017, Journal of Neuroscience, Vol. 37, pp. 464-473.

211. **Poe, Gina, [perf.].** Use Sleep to Enhance Memory, Learning, and Emotional State. [comps.] Huberman Lab. 2023.

212. *Links between the brain and body during sleep: implications for memory processing.* **Whitehurst, L.N., et al.** 1783, 2021, Trends in Neurosciences.

213. *Corticosteroids: the drugs to beat.* **Barnes, P.J.** 1-3, s.l. : Eur J Pharmacol., 2006, Vol. 533, pp. 2-14.

214. *Chronic stress, cortisol dysfunction, and pain: a psychoneuroendocrine rationale for stress management in pain rehabilitation.* **Hannibal, K.E. and Bishop, M.D.** 12, s.l. : Phys Ther., 2014, Vol. 94, pp. 1816-25.

215. *Mitochondrial allostatic load puts the 'gluc' back in glucocorticoids.* **Picard, M., Juster, R. P. and McEwen, B. S.** 5, 2014, Nature Reviews Endocrinology, Vol. 10, pp. 303-310.

216. *Mechanisms linking obesity to insulin resistance and type 2 diabetes.* **Kahn, S. E., Hull, R. L. and Utzschneider, K. M.** 7121, 2006, Nature, Vol. 444, pp. 840-846.

217. *Oxidative stress and diabetic complications.* **Giacco, F. and Brownlee, M.** 9, 2010, Circulation Research, Vol. 107, pp. 1058-1070.

218. *Normalizing mitochondrial superoxide production blocks three pathways of hyperglycaemic damage.* **Nishikawa, T., et al.** 6779, 2000, Nature, Vol. 404, pp. 787-790.

219. *Actions of corticosterone on the oxidative stress in rat hippocampal neurons.* **Liu, J., et al.** 10, 2000, Life Sciences, Vol. 67, pp. 1195-1205.

220. *Urinary cortisol and six-year risk of all-cause and cardiovascular mortality.* **Vogelzangs, N., et al.** 11, 2014, Journal of Clinical Endocrinology & Metabolism, Vol. 95, pp. 4959-4964.

221. *Current Directions in Stress and Human Immune Function.* **Morey, J.N., et al.** s.l. : Curr Opin Psychol., 2015, Vol. 5, pp. 13-17.

222. *Glutamate: The Master Neurotransmitter and Its Implications in Chronic Stress and Mood Disorders.* **Pal, M.M.** 2021, Front Hum Neurosci., Vol. 15.

223. *Glucocorticoids and hippocampal atrophy in neuropsychiatric disorders.* **Sapolsky, R. M.** 10, 2000, Archives of General Psychiatry, Vol. 57, pp. 925-935.

224. *Mitochondrial DNA damage as a mechanism of oxidative stress in rheumatoid arthritis.* **Sander, M., Sander, M. and Hayes, G.** 4, 2007, Nature Reviews Rheumatology, Vol. 3, pp. 237-242.

225. *The Relation Between Adverse Childhood Experiences and Adult Health: Turning Gold into Lead.* **Felitti, V.J.** 1, 2002, The Permanente Journal, Vol. 6, pp. 44–47.

226. **Mate, G.** *In the Realm of Hungry Ghosts: Close Encounters with Addiction.* s.l. : Random House, 2018.

227. *Examining Perceived Stress, Childhood Trauma and Interpersonal Trauma in Individuals With Drug Addiction.* **Garami, J., et al.** 2, 2019, Psychological Reports, Vol. 122, pp. 433-450.

228. *How Emotions Develop and How they Organise Development.* **Fischer, K. W., Shaver, P. R. and Carnochan, P.** 2, 1990, Cognition and Emotion, Vol. 4, pp. 81–127.

229. **Johnstone, L. and Boyle, M.** *Power Threat Meaning Framework.* s.l. : The British Psychological Society, 2018.

230. *he Enteric Nervous System and Its Emerging Role as a Therapeutic Target.* **Fleming, M.A. 2nd, et al.** 8024171, 2020, Gastroenterol Res Pract.

231. **Ancestry Foundation.** Lifestyle and Autoimmune Disease — Sarah Ballantyne, Ph.D. (AHS14). *YouTube.* [Online] 24th August 2014. https://www.youtube.com/watch?v=02szpuypkOg.

232. *Mechanisms of Intestinal Barrier Dysfunction in Sepsis.* **Yoseph, B.P., et al.** 1, s.l. : Shock, 2016, Vol. 46.

233. *Tight junctions, intestinal permeability, and autoimmunity: celiac disease and type 1 diabetes paradigms.* **Visser J, Rozing J, Sapone A, Lammers K, Fasano A.** 2009, Ann N Y Acad Sci., Vol. 1165, pp. 195-205.

234. *Nonceliac gluten sensitivity.* **Fasano, A., et al.** 6, 2015, Gastroenterology, Vol. 148, pp. 1195-1204.e4.

235. *Changes in intestinal tight junction permeability associated with industrial food additives explain the rising incidence of autoimmune disease.* **Lerner, A. and Matthias, T.** 6, 2015, Autoimmun Rev, Vol. 14, pp. 479-489.

236. *Highly Efficient Gluten Degradation by Lactobacilli and Fungal Proteases during Food Processing: New Perspectives for Celiac Disease.* **Rizzello CG, De Angelis M, Di Cagno R, Camarca, A., et al.** 2007, Appl Environ Microbiol, Vol. 73.

237. *Assessing the efficacy of oral immunotherapy for the desensitisation of peanut allergy in children (STOP II): a phase 2 randomised controlled trial.* **Anagnostou, K. and et al.** 9925, 2014, The Lancet, Vol. 383, pp. 1297-1304.

238. *Oxidative stress in humans during work at moderate altitude.* **Gomes, L. F. and et al.** 1, 2018, Journal of Physiological Anthropology, Vol. 37, p. 8.

239. **Sanchez-Muniz, F. J. and Bastida, S.** Fruits as dietary sources of sugars and antioxidants. *Antioxidants in food: Practical applications.* s.l. : Woodhead Publishing, 2012, pp. 243-267.

240. **Serafini, M. and et al.** Redox regulation of cardiovascular function. *Antioxidant measurement and applications.* s.l. : ACOS Press, 2010, pp. 219-237.

241. *Free radicals, antioxidants and functional foods: Impact on human health.* **Lobo, V. and et al.** 8, 2010, Pharmacognosy Reviews, Vol. 4, pp. 118-126.

242. *Dietary emulsifiers impact the mouse gut microbiota promoting colitis and metabolic syndrome.* **Chassaing, B. and et al.** 7541, 2017, Nature, Vol. 519, pp. 92-96.

243. **Huberman Lab.** Dr. Robert Lustig: How Sugar & Processed Foods Impact Your Health. *YouTube.* [Online] 19th December 2023. https://www.youtube.com/watch?v=n28W4AmvMDE.

244. **National Research Council (US) Subcommittee on the Tenth Edition of the Recommended Dietary Allowances.** *Protein and amino acids.* s.l. : National Academies Press, 1989.

245. **Harper, D.** Online Etymology Dictionary. [Online] https://www.etymonline.com/.

246. *Nutritional modulation of immune function.* **Grimble, R. F.** 3, 2001, Proceedings of the Nutrition Society, Vol. 60, pp. 389-397.

247. *The role of protein and amino acids in immune function.* **Samman, S. and & Sriram, K.** 2, 1997, American Journal of Clinical Nutrition, Vol. 66, pp. 579S-585S.

248. *Evidence-based pharmacotherapy of generalized anxiety disorder.* **Baldwin, D. S. and Polkinghorn, C.** 2, 2005, International Journal of Neuropsychopharmacology, Vol. 8, pp. 293-302.

249. *History and evolution of the monoamine hypothesis of depression.* **Hirschfeld, R. M.** 6, 4-6, Journal of Clinical Psychiatry, Vol. 61, pp. 4-6.

250. *Targeting the murine serotonin transporter: insights into human neurobiology.* **Murphy, D. L. and Lesch, K. P.** 2008, Nature Reviews Neuroscience, Vol. 92, pp. 85-96.

251. *Serotonin and Anxiolytic Properties of SSRIs.* **Argyropoulos, S. V. and Nutt, D. J.** 4, 2000, Journal of Clinical Psychiatry, Vol. 61, pp. 24-30.

252. **Huberman Lab.** Dr. Diego Bohórquez: The Science of Your Gut Sense & the Gut-Brain Axis. [Online] 27th May 2024. https://www.hubermanlab.com/episode/dr-diego-bohorquez-the-science-of-your-gut-sense-the-gut-brain-axis.

253. *Testing Protein Leverage in Lean Humans: A Randomised Controlled Experimental Study.* **Gosby, A.K., et al.** 10, 2011, PLOS ONE, Vol. 6.

254. *Effects of prenatal protein malnutrition on the hippocampal formation.* **Morgane, P.J., Mokler, D.J. and Galler, J.R.** 4, 2002, Neuroscience & Biobehavioral Reviews, Vol. 26, pp. 471-483.

255. *Effects of 30 days of undernutrition on plasma neurotransmitter precursors, other amino acids, and behavior.* **Liebermen, H.R., et al.** 3, 1997, Effects of 30 days of undernutrition on plasma neurotransmitter precursors, other amino acids, and behavior, Vol. 8, pp. 119-126.

256. *The role of protein and amino acids in immune function.* **Samman, S. and Sriram, K.** 2, 1997, American Journal of Clinical Nutrition, Vol. 66, pp. 579S-585S.

257. *The role of the sensory systems in the immune response and autoimmune diseases.* **Nisticò, R., Coppedè, F. and**

Falvo, F. 3, 2018, Clinical Reviews in Allergy & Immunology, Vol. 54, pp. 364-380.

258. *Toward a new recommended dietary allowance for vitamin C based on antioxidant and health effects in humans.* **Carr, A. and Frei, B.** 6, 1999, The American Journal of Clinical Nutrition, Vol. 69, pp. 1086-1107.

259. *Vitamin E: function and metabolism.* **Brigelius-Flohé, R. and Traber, M. G.** 10, 1999, The FASEB Journal, Vol. 13, pp. 1145-1155.

260. *Polyphenols: antioxidants and beyond.* **Scalbert, A., Johnson, I. T. and Saltmarsh, M.** 1, 2005, The American Journal of Clinical Nutrition, Vol. 81, pp. 215S-217S.

261. *The changing faces of glutathione, a cellular protagonist.* **Pompella, A., et al.** 8, 2003, Biochemical Pharmacology, Vol. 66, pp. 1499-1503.

262. *Diversity of structures and properties among catalases.* **Chelikani, P., Fita, I. and Loewen, P. C.** 2, 2004, Cellular and Molecular Life Sciences, Vol. 61, pp. 192-208.

263. *Superoxide dismutase. An enzymic function for erythrocuprein (hemocuprein).* **McCord, J. M. and Fridovich, I.** 22, 1969, The Journal of Biological Chemistry, Vol. 244, pp. 6049-6055.

264. *Dietary reference intakes for energy, carbohydrate, fiber, fat, fatty acids, cholesterol, protein, and amino acids.* **National Academies of Sciences, Engineering, and Medicine.** 2020, The National Academies Press.

265. *The amino acid requirements of adult man.* **Rose, W. C.** 9, 1957, Nutrition Reviews, Vol. 15, pp. 289-300.

266. *Evidence-based recommendations for optimal dietary protein intake in older people: a position paper from the PROT-AGE Study Group.* **Bauer, J., et al.** 8, 2013, Journal of the American Medical Directors Association, Vol. 14, pp. 542-559.

267. *Long-term testosterone gel (Androgel) treatment maintains beneficial effects on sexual function and mood, lean body mass, and muscle strength, and decreases visceral fat in hypogonadal men.* **Wang, C., et al.** 8, 1996, Journal of

Clinical Endocrinology and Metabolism, Vol. 85, pp. 2839-2853.

268. *Appropriate protein provision in critical illness: a systematic and narrative review.* **Hoffer, L. J. and Bistrian, B. R.** 6, 2013, American Journal of Clinical Nutrition, Vol. 98, pp. 989-1002.

269. *Physical performance and metabolic changes induced by combined prolonged exercise and different energy intakes in humans.* **Guezennec, C. Y., et al.** 7, 1989, European Journal of Applied Physiology and Occupational Physiology, Vol. 58, pp. 699-704.

270. *Essential amino acids are primarily responsible for the amino acid stimulation of muscle protein anabolism in healthy elderly adults.* **Volpi, E., et al.** 2, 2001, American Journal of Clinical Nutrition, Vol. 73, pp. 647-656.

271. *Inverse regulation of protein turnover and amino acid transport in skeletal muscle of septic patients.* **Biolo, G., Fleming, R. Y. and Maggi, S. P.** 6, 1997, Journal of Clinical Investigation, Vol. 99, pp. 1408-1417.

272. *Dietary protein requirements in athletes.* **Lemon, P.W.R.** 2, 1997, The Journal of Nutritional Biochemistry, Vol. 8, pp. 52-60.

273. **Sims, S. T. and Fitzgerald, C.** *Roar: How to Match Your Food and Fitness to Your Unique Female Physiology for Optimum Performance, Great Health, and a Strong, Lean Body for Life.* s.l. : Rodale Books, 2023.

274. *A systematic review, meta-analysis and meta-regression of the effect of protein supplementation on resistance training-induced gains in muscle mass and strength in healthy adults.* **Morton, R. W., et al.** 6, s.l. : British Journal of Sports Medicine, 2018, Vol. 55, pp. 376-384.

275. *One-carbon metabolism–genome interactions in folate-associated pathologies.* **Stover, P. J.** 12, 2009, The Journal of Nutrition, Vol. 139, pp. 2402-2405.

276. *Muscle adenylate deaminase deficiency.* **Argov, Z., et al.** 1, 1981, Archives of Neurology, Vol. 38, pp. 456-460.

277. *Current concepts and unresolved questions in dietary protein requirements and supplements in adults.* **Phillips, S. M.** 13, 2017, Frontiers in Nutrition, Vol. 4.

278. *Characterising the muscle anabolic potential of dairy, meat and plant-based protein sources in older adults.* **Gorissen, S. H. and Witard, O. C.** 1, 2018, Proceedings of the Nutrition Society, Vol. 77, pp. 20-31.

279. **Merrill, A. L., & Watt, B. K.** *Energy value of foods: Basis and derivation.* s.l. : U.S. Department of Agriculture, Agricultural Research Service, 1973.

280. *International Society of Sports Nutrition Position Stand: protein and exercise.* **Jäger, R., et al.** 20, 2017, J Int Soc Sports Nutr, Vol. 14.

281. *Nutrient intakes and food sources of rugby players: A systematic review.* **Ball, L. and Ackland, T. R.** 1, 2020, Journal of the International Society of Sports Nutrition, Vol. 17.

282. *Content of free amino acids in buckwheat (Fagopyrum esculentum Moench) seeds, seedlings and plants at different growth stages.* **Bonafaccia, G., et al.** 3, 2003, Journal of Food Composition and Analysis, Vol. 16, pp. 343-354.

283. *Hempseed as a nutritional resource: An overview.* **Callaway, J. C.** 1-2, 2004, Euphytica, Vol. 140, pp. 65-72.

284. *Soy and health update: Evaluation of the clinical and epidemiologic literature.* **Messina, M.** 12, 2016, Nutrients, Vol. 8, p. 754.

285. *lavonoids and other phenolic compounds in Andean indigenous grains: Quinoa (Chenopodium quinoa), kaniwa (Chenopodium pallidicaule) and kiwicha (Amaranthus caudatus).* **Repo-Carrasco-Valencia, R., et al.** 1, 2010, Food Chemistry, Vol. 120, pp. 128-133.

286. *Supplementation of conventional therapy with the novel grain Salba (Salvia hispanica L.) improves major and emerging cardiovascular risk factors in type 2 diabetes: Results of a randomized controlled trial.* **Vuksan, V., et al.** 2, 2010, Diabetes Care, Vol. 33, pp. 250-251.

287. *A Review of Dietary (Phyto)Nutrients for Glutathione Support.* **Minnich, D.M. and Brown, B.I.** 9, 2019, Nutrients, Vol. 11.

288. *Glutathione: a key player in autoimmunity.* **Perricone, C, De Carolis, C. and Perricone, R.** 8, 2009, Autoimmun Rev., Vol. 8, pp. 697-701.

289. *Effects of cooking on rutin and glutathione concentrations and antioxidant activity of green asparagus (Asparagus officinalis) spears.* **Drinkwater, J.M., et al.** 2015, Journal of Functional Foods, Vol. 12, pp. 342-353.

290. **WHO.** Cardiovascular diseases. [Online] https://www.who.int/health-topics/cardiovascular-diseases#tab=tab_1.

291. **Teicholz, N.** *The Big Fat Surprise: Why Butter, Meat and Cheese Belong in a Healthy Diet.* s.l. : Simon & Schuster, 2014.

292. **WHO.** Replace Trans Fat. [Online] 1 May 2018. https://www.who.int/docs/default-source/documents/replace-transfats/replace-act-information-sheet.pdf.

293. *Balancing cholesterol synthesis and absorption in the gastrointestinal tract.* **Cohen, D.E.** 2, s.l. : J Clin Lipidol., 2008, Vol. 2, pp. S1-3.

294. *Differences in Response to Egg Intake Result in Distinct Lipoprotein Profiles While Plasma Concentrations of Carotenoids and Choline Are Not Affected.* **Fernandez, M.L. and DiMarco, D.** Supp 1, s.l. : Curr Dev Nutr., 2019, Vol. 3, pp. 102-19.

295. **National Institutes of Health.** *Dietary Fats.* [Online] 2020. https://www.nih.gov/.

296. *Treatments of low rank coals for improved power generation and reduction in Greenhouse gas emissions.* **Domazetis, G., et al.** 1, 2008, Fuel Processing Technology, Vol. 89, pp. 68-76.

297. **Nelson, D. L. and Cox, M. M.** *Lehninger Principles of Biochemistry (5th ed.).* s.l. : W.H. Freeman., 2008.

298. **Brooks, G. A., Fahey, T. D. and Baldwin, K. M.** *Exercise Physiology: Human Bioenergetics and Its Applications (4th ed.).* s.l. : McGraw-Hill Education, 2005.

299. **McArdle, W. D., Katch, F. I. and Katch, V. L.** *Exercise Physiology: Nutrition, Energy, and Human Performance (7th ed.).* s.l. : Wolters Kluwer Health, 2010.

300. *The importance of the ratio of omega-6/omega-3 essential fatty acids.* **Simopoulos, A. P.** 8, 2002, Biomedicine & Pharmacotherapy, Vol. 56, pp. 365-379.

301. *n-3 Fatty acids and inflammation: From molecular biology to the clinic.* **Calder, P. C.** 3, 2006, Biological Reviews, Vol. 81, pp. 435-457.

302. *The Sources, Synthesis and Biological Actions of Omega-3 and Omega-6 Fatty Acids in Red Meat: An Overview.* **Ponnampalam, E.N., Sinclair, A.J. and Holman, B.W.B.** 6, 2021, Foods, Vol. 10.

303. *Alpha-linolenic acid and its conversion to longer chain n−3 fatty acids: Benefits for human health and a role in maintaining tissue n−3 fatty acid levels.* **Barceló-Coblijn, G. and Murphy, E.J.** 6, 2009, Progress in Lipid Research, Vol. 48, pp. 355-374.

304. *Extra Virgin Olive Oil Extracts of Indigenous Southern Tuscany Cultivar Act as Anti-Inflammatory and Vasorelaxant Nutraceuticals.* **Pozzetti, L., et al.** 3, 2022, Antioxidants, Vol. 11.

305. *Chemistry and Functionality of Cold-Pressed Macadamia Nut Oil.* **Kaseke, T., Fwole, O.A. and Opara, U.L.** 1, 2022, Processes, Vol. 10.

306. **Battula, S.N., et al.** Ghee, Anhydrous Milk Fat and Butteroil. [book auth.] T. Truong, et al. *Dairy Fat Products and Functionality.* s.l. : Springer, 2020, pp. 399-430.

307. *Macadamia nut oil: A healthful addition to your diet.* **McDaniel, M. A., Maier, S. F. and Einstein, G. O.** 5, 2012, Journal of Food Science, Vol. 77, pp. R75-R85.

308. *Nutritional and health aspects of avocado oil.* **Berglund, L., Lu, Y. and Hernandez, L. M.** 7, 2014,

Critical Reviews in Food Science and Nutrition, Vol. 54, pp. 762-770.

309. *Mechanisms for insulin resistance: Common threads and missing links.* **Samuel, V. T. and Shulman, G. I.** 5, 2016, Cell, Vol. 148, pp. 852-871.

310. *Hypoxia is a potential risk factor for chronic inflammation and adiponectin reduction in adipose tissue of obese subjects.* **Ye, J., et al.** 8, 2007, Obesity, Vol. 15, pp. 1640-1645.

311. *Pathophysiology of sex hormone binding globulin (SHBG): relation to insulin.* **Pugeat, M., et al.** 4-6, 1991, Journal of Steroid Biochemistry and Molecular Biology, Vol. 40, pp. 841-849.

312. *Reproductive hormones and the menopause transition.* **Santoro, N. and Randolph Jr, J. F.** 3, 2011, Obstetrics and Gynecology Clinics, Vol. 38, pp. 455-466.

313. **Delgado, B.J. and Lopez-Ojeda, W.** Statpearls: Estrogen. *National Library of Medicine.* [Online] 26th June 2023. https://www.ncbi.nlm.nih.gov/books/NBK538260/.

314. *Sex Hormones in Acquired Immunity and Autoimmune Disease.* **Moulton, V.R.** 9, 2018, Front Immunol.

315. **Poretsky, L.** *Principles of diabetes mellitus.* s.l. : Springer Science & Business Media, 2010.

316. *Hypoglycemia, but not insulin, acutely decreases LH and T secretion in men.* **Oltmanns, K.M., et al.** 10, s.l. : J Clin Endocrinol Metab., 2001, Vol. 86.

317. *The molecular biology, biochemistry, and physiology of human steroidogenesis and its disorders.* **Miller, W.L. and Auchus, R.J.** 1, s.l. : Endocr Rev., 2011, Vol. 32, pp. 81-151.

318. *Hypothalamic-pituitary-adrenal axis, neuroendocrine factors and stress.* **Tsigos, C. and Chrousos, G. P.** 4, 2002, Journal of Psychosomatic Research, Vol. 53, pp. 865-871.

319. *Deiodinases: Implications of the local control of thyroid hormone action.* **Bianco, A. C. and Kim, B. W.** 10, 2006, Journal of Clinical Investigation, Vol. 116, pp. 2571-2579.

320. *Gender differences in substrate for endurance exercise.* **Tarnopolsky, L.J., et al.** 1, 1985, J Appl Physiol, Vol. 68, pp. 302-8.

321. *Smaller muscle ATP reduction in women than in men by repeated bouts of sprint exercise.* **Esbjörnsson-Liljedahl, M., Bodin, K. and E., Jansson.** 3, 1985, J Appl Physiol, Vol. 93, pp. 1075-83.

322. *Sex differences in exercise metabolism and the role of 17-beta estradiol.* **Tarnopolsky, M.A.** 4, 2008, Med Sci Sports Exerc., Vol. 40, pp. 648-54.

323. *A reduced ratio of dietary carbohydrate to protein improves body composition and blood lipid profiles during weight loss in adult women.* **Layman, D. K., et al.** 2, 2003, The Journal of Nutrition, Vol. 133, pp. 411-417.

324. *The Canadian Trial of Carbohydrates in Diabetes (CCD), a 1-year controlled trial of low-glycemic-index dietary carbohydrate in type 2 diabetes: no effect on glycated hemoglobin but reduction in C-reactive protein.* **Wolever, T. M. S., et al.** 3, 2009, The American Journal of Clinical Nutrition, Vol. 90, pp. 517-524.

325. *Control of blood glucose in type 2 diabetes without weight loss by modification of diet composition.* **Gannon, M.C. and Nuttall, F.Q.** 16, 2006, Nutrition & Metabolism, Vol. 3.

326. *HPLC Determination of Folate in Liver and Liver Products.* **Vahteristo, L., Ollilainen, V. and Varo, P.** 3, 1996, Food Science, Vol. 61, pp. 524-526.

327. *Beef as a source of bioactive components.* **Sadowska, A., et al.** 2014, Zeszyty Problemowe Postępów Nauk Rolniczych, Vol. 576, pp. 121–130.

328. **Gropper, S. S., Smith, J. L. and Carr, T. P.** *Advanced Nutrition and Human Metabolism (7th ed.).* s.l. : Cengage Learning, 2017.

329. **Whitney, E. N., et al.** *Understanding Nutrition: Australian and New Zealand Edition (2nd ed.).* s.l. : Cengage Learning Australia, 2016.

330. *Mercury Exposure and Antinuclear Antibodies among Females of Reproductive Age in the United States: NHANES.* **Somers, E.C., et al.** 8, s.l. : Environ Health Perspect., 2015, Vol. 123.

331. *Functional consequence of Iron dyshomeostasis and ferroptosis in systemic lupus erythematosus and lupus nephritis.* **Morel, L. and Scindia, Y.** s.l. : Clin Immunol., 2024, Vol. 262.

332. *Immunomodulation by heavy metals as a contributing factor to inflammatory diseases and autoimmune reactions: Cadmium as an example.* **Aleksandrove, A.P. and et al. .** s.l. : Immunology Letters, 2021, Vol. 240, pp. 106-122.

333. *Modulation of Metabolic Detoxification Pathways Using Foods and Food-Derived Components: A Scientific Review with Clinical Application.* **Hodges, R.E. and Minich, D.M.** 2015, J Nutr Metab. .

334. *Iron deficiency and iron excess damage mitochondria and mitochondrial DNA in rats.* **Walter, P.B., et al.** 4, s.l. : PNAS, 2002, Vol. 99, pp. 2264-2269 .

335. *Dietary Micronutrient Management to Treat Mitochondrial Dysfunction in Diet-Induced Obese Mice.* **Cimmino, F., et al.** 6, s.l. : International Journal of Molecular Sciences, 2021, Vol. 22.

336. **National Institutes of Health.** Vitamin D Fact Sheet for Health Professionals. [Online] 2021. https://ods.od.nih.gov/factsheets/VitaminD-HealthProfessional.

337. *The role of vitamin D in autoimmune diseases: could sex make the difference?* **Dupuis, M.L., et al.** 2, 2021, Biol Sex Differ, Vol. 12.

338. *Vitamin D as a Nutri-Epigenetic Factor in Autoimmunity-A Review of Current Research and Reports on Vitamin D Deficiency in Autoimmune Diseases.* **Mazur, A., Frączek, P. and Tabarkiewicz, J.** 20, s.l. : Nutrients, 2022, Vol. 14.

339. **Berg, E.D.** Fascinating Insights on Hashimoto's (Hypothyroidism). *YouTube.* [Online] 12th April 2024. https://www.youtube.com/watch?v=fl7DU7-wfv0.

340. *Vitamin D and intestinal calcium absorption.* **Christakos, S., et al.** 1-2, s.l. : Mol Cell Endocrinol., 2011, Vol. 347, pp. 25-9.

341. **Campbell, J.** Vitamin D doses. *YouTube.* [Online] 16th May 2023. https://www.youtube.com/watch?v=E3_t-EQIy0s.

342. **National Instutes of Health.** Vitamin D. [Online] 18th September 2023. https://ods.od.nih.gov/factsheets/VitaminD-HealthProfessional/#:~:text=RDAs%20for%20vitamin%20D%20are,40%20IU%20(Table%202)..

343. *A Narrative Review of the Evidence for Variations in Serum 25-Hydroxyvitamin D Concentration Thresholds for Optimal Health.* **Grant, W.B., et al.** 3, 2022, Nutrients, Vol. 14.

344. *Estimates of optimal vitamin D status.* **Dawson-Hughes, B., et al.** 7, s.l. : Osteoporos Int., 2005, Vol. 16, pp. 713-6.

345. *Omega-3 fatty acids and inflammatory processes: from molecules to man.* **Calder, P. C.** 5, 2017, Biochemical Society Transactions, Vol. 45, pp. 1105-1115.

346. *Critical review: vegetables and fruit in the prevention of chronic diseases.* **Boeing, H., et al.** 6, 2012, European Journal of Nutrition, Vol. 51, pp. 637-663.

347. *Health-promoting components of fruits and vegetables in the diet.* **Liu, R. H.** 3, 2013, Advances in Nutrition, Vol. 4, pp. 384S-392S.

348. *Dysbiosis in Inflammatory Bowel Disease: Pathogenic Role and Potential Therapeutic Targets.* **Santana, P.T., et al.** s.l. : Int. J. Mol. Sci, 2022, Vol. 23. 3464.

349. *A clinician's primer on the role of the microbiome in human health and disease.* **Khanna, S. and Tosh, P.K.** 1, s.l. : Mayo Clin Proc., 2014, Vol. 89.

350. *The Gut Microbiome, Aging, and Longevity: A Systematic Review.* **Badal, V.D., et al.** 12, 2020, Nutrients, Vol. 12.

351. *Dietary fiber and body weight.* **Slavin, J. L.** 3, 2013, Nutrition, Vol. 21, pp. 411-418.

352. **Rengel, Z.** *Handbook of soil acidity.* s.l. : CRC Press, 2002.

353. *Vitamin D deficiency in Europe: Pandemic?* **Cashman, K. D. and Dowling, K. G.** 4, 2014, The American Journal of Clinical Nutrition, Vol. 103, pp. 1033-1044.

354. *The prevalence of cobalamin deficiency among vegetarians assessed by serum vitamin B12: A review of literature.* **Pawlak, R., Lester, S. E. and Babatunde, T.** 5, 2013, European Journal of Clinical Nutrition, Vol. 68, pp. 541-548.

355. *Vitamin D deficiency.* **Holick, M. F.** 3, 2007, New England Journal of Medicine, Vol. 357, pp. 266-281.

356. *Achieving optimal essential fatty acid status in vegetarians: Current knowledge and practical implications.* **Davis, B. C. and Kris-Etherton, P. M.** 3, 2003, The American Journal of Clinical Nutrition, Vol. 78, pp. 640S-646S.

357. *Are all n-3 polyunsaturated fatty acids created equal?* **Anderson, B.M. and Ma, D.W.** 33, s.l. : Lipids Health Dis., 2009, Vol. 8.

358. *Iron bioavailability and dietary reference values.* **Hurrell, R. and Egli, I.** 5, 2010, The American Journal of Clinical Nutrition, Vol. 91, pp. 1461S-1467S.

359. *Position of the Academy of Nutrition and Dietetics: Vegetarian diets.* **Melina, V., Craig, W. and Levin, S.** 12, 2016, Journal of the Academy of Nutrition and Dietetics, Vol. 116, pp. 1970-1980.

360. *Use of creatine in the elderly and evidence for effects on cognitive function in young and old.* **Rawson, E. S. and Venezia, A. C.** 5, 2011, Amino Acids, Vol. 40, pp. 1349-1362.

361. *International Society of Sports Nutrition position stand: Safety and efficacy of creatine supplementation in exercise, sport, and medicine.* **Kreider, R. B., et al.** 18, 2017, Journal of the International Society of Sports Nutrition, Vol. 14.

362. *Creatine supplementation with specific view to exercise/sports performance: An update.* **Cooper, R., et al.** 1, 2012, Journal of the International Society of Sports Nutrition, Vol. 9.

363. *Creatine in the elderly and patients with muscle-wasting diseases: A review.* **Sakkas, G. K.** 6, 2014, European Journal of Nutrition, Vol. 53, pp. 1313-1328.

364. *Long-term creatine supplementation is safe in aged patients with Parkinson disease.* **Bender, A., et al.** 4, 2008, Nutritional Neuroscience, Vol. 11, pp. 172-176.

365. *Use of creatine in the elderly and evidence for effects on cognitive function in young and old.* **Rawson, E. S. and Venezia, A. C.** 5, 2011, Amino Acids, Vol. 40, pp. 1349-1362.

366. *Microbes and mental health: a review.* **Rieder, R., Wisniewski, P. J., Alderman, B. L., & Campbell, S. C.** 2017, Brain, Behavior, and Immunity, Vol. 66, pp. 9-17.

367. *Exercise-induced stress behavior, gut-microbiota-brain axis and diet: a systematic review for athletes.* **Clark, A. and Mach, N.** 1, 2016, Journal of the International Society of Sports Nutrition, Vol. 13, p. 43.

368. *Role of the microbiota in immunity and inflammation.* **Belkaid, Y. and Hand, T. W.** 1, 2014, Cell, Vol. 157, pp. 121-141.

369. *The microbiota in adaptive immune homeostasis and disease.* **Honda, K. and Littman, D. R.** 7610, 2016, Nature, Vol. 535, pp. 75-84.

370. *From dietary fiber to host physiology: short-chain fatty acids as key bacterial metabolites.* **Koh, A., et al.** 6, 2016, Cell, Vol. 165, pp. 1332-1345.

371. *Leaky gut and autoimmune diseases.* **Fasano, A.** 1, 2012, Clinical Reviews in Allergy & Immunology, Vol. 42, pp. 71-78.

372. *he gut microbiota shapes intestinal immune responses during health and disease.* **Round, J. L. and Mazmanian, S. K.** 5, 2009, Nature Reviews Immunology, Vol. 9, pp. 313-323.

373. *The microbiome and innate immunity.* **Thaiss, C. A., et al.** 7610, 2016, Nature, Vol. 535, pp. 65-74.

374. *Induction of colonic regulatory T cells by indigenous Clostridium species.* **Atarashi, K., et al.** 6015, 2011, Science, Vol. 331, pp. 337-341.

375. *Diet-Microbiome Interactions in Health Are Controlled by Intestinal Nitrogen Source Constraints.* **Holmes, A.J., et al.** 1, 2017, Cell Metab., Vol. 25, pp. 140-151.

376. *Influence of diet on the gut microbiome and implications for human health.* **Singh, R.K., et al.** 1, 2017, J Transl Med., Vol. 15.

377. **USDA.** FoodData Central. [Online] 2019. https://fdc.nal.usda.gov.

378. *Chemical composition and microflora of black cumin (Nigella sativa L.) seeds growing in Saudi Arabia.* **Al-Jassir, M.S.** 4, s.l. : Food Chemistry, 1992, Vol. 45.

379. *Fasting: Molecular Mechanisms and Clinical Applications.* **Longo, V. D. and Mattson, M. P.** 2, 2014, Cell Metabolism, Vol. 19, p. Cell Metabolism.

380. *Autophagy fights disease through cellular self-digestion.* **Mizushima, N., et al.** 7182, 2008, Nature, Vol. 451, pp. 1069-1075.

381. *Mechanisms of mitophagy.* **Youle, R. J. and Narendra, D. P.** 1, 2011, Nature Reviews Molecular Cell Biology, Vol. 12, pp. 9-14.

382. *PGC-1α, SIRT1 and AMPK, an energy sensing network that controls energy expenditure.* **Cantó, C. and Auwerx, J.** 2, 2009, Current Opinion in Lipidology, Vol. 20, pp. 98-105.

383. *Calorie restriction induces mitochondrial biogenesis and bioenergetic efficiency.* **López-Lluch, G., et al.** 6, 2006, Proceedings of the National Academy of Sciences, Vol. 103, pp. 1768-1773.

384. *SIRT1 exerts anti-inflammatory effects and improves insulin sensitivity in adipocytes.* **Yoshizaki, T., et al.** 5, 2009, Molecular and Cellular Biology, Vol. 29, pp. 1363-1374.

385. *Acetylation-deacetylation of the transcription factor Nrf2 (NF-E2-related factor 2) regulates its transcriptional activity and nucleocytoplasmic localization.* **Kawai, Y., et al.** 9, 2011, Journal of Biological Chemistry, Vol. 286, pp. 7629-7640.

386. *Cell survival responses to environmental stresses via the Keap1-Nrf2-ARE pathway.* **Kensler, T. W., Wakabayashi, N. and Biswal, S.** 2007, Annual Review of Pharmacology and Toxicology, Vol. 47, pp. 89-116.

387. *Resveratrol-activated SIRT1 in liver and pancreas.* **Vetterli, L. and Maechler, P.** 10, 2011, Biochimica et Biophysica Acta (BBA)-General Subjects, Vol. 1810, pp. 1075-1086.

388. *Lessons from C. elegans: Signaling pathways for longevity.* **Lapierre, L. R. and Hansen, M.** 12, 2012, Trends in Endocrinology & Metabolism, Vol. 23, pp. 637-644.

389. *Flipping the Metabolic Switch: Understanding and Applying the Health Benefits of Fasting.* **Anton, S. D., et al.** 12, 2015, Obesity, Vol. 23, pp. 2322–2330.

390. *Extending the Overnight Fast: Sex Differences in Acute Metabolic Responses to Breakfast.* **S. Atkinson, F., et al.** 8, 2020, Nutrients, Vol. 12.

391. *Intermittent and periodic fasting, longevity and disease.* **Longo, V.D., et al.** 2021, Nature Aging, Vol. 1, pp. 47–59.

392. *Fasting-Mimicking Diet Promotes Ngn3-Driven β-Cell Regeneration to Reverse Diabetes.* **Cheng, C.W., et al.** 5, 2017, Cell, Vol. 168, pp. 775-788.E12.

393. *Exposure to Environmental Toxins and Autoimmune Conditions.* **Kharrazian, D.** 2, 2021, Integr Med, Vol. 20, pp. 20-24.

394. *Kalofiri, P.; Biskanaki, F.; Kefala, V.; Tertipi, N.; Sfyri, E.; Rallis, E.* **Kalofiri, P., et al.** 3, 2023, Cosmetics, Vol. 10.

395. *Identification of combinations of endocrine disrupting chemicals in household chemical products that require mixture toxicity testing.* **Lee, I. and Ji, K.** 2022, Ecotoxicol Environ Saf., Vol. 240.

396. **EWG.** Glyphosate Contamination in Food Goes Far Beyond Oat Products. [Online] 2019. https://www.ewg.org/news-insights/news/2019/02/glyphosate-contamination-food-goes-far-beyond-oat-products.

397. **CDC.** Air Pollutants. [Online] https://www.cdc.gov/air-quality/pollutants/?CDC_AAref_Val=https://www.cdc.gov/air/pollutants.htm.

398. *Bisphenol S and F: A systematic review and comparison of the hormonal activity of bisphenol A substitutes.* **Rochester, J. R. and Bolden, A. L.** 7, 2015, Environmental Health Perspectives, Vol. 123, pp. 643-650.

399. *Chronic exposure to phthalates increases reactive oxygen species production in rat hearts, but attenuates ischemia/reperfusion injury following ischemia pretreatment.* **Sharma, A. and Hu, Y.** 8, 2019, The Journal of Toxicological Sciences, Vol. 44, pp. 551-561.

400. *Stapled peptides inhibitors of RAS.* **Pillai, H. K., et al.** 9-10, 2015, Biological Chemistry, Vol. 396, pp. 1005-1016.

401. *Brain-inhabiting bacteria and neurodegenerative diseases: the "brain microbiome" theory.* **Arabi, T.Z., et al.** 2023, Front. Aging Neurosci., Vol. 15.

402. *Hay fever, hygiene, and household size.* **Strachan, D. P.** 6710, 1989, BMJ, Vol. 299, pp. 1259-1260.

403. **Simon, M.** *A Poison Like No Other: How Microplastics Corrupted Our Planet and Our Bodies.* s.l. : Island Press, 2022.

404. *Endocrine disruptors and asthma-associated chemicals in consumer products.* **Dodson, R. E., et al.** 7, 2012, Environmental Health Perspectives, Vol. 120, pp. 935-943.

405. *Endocrine disruptors and human health: could oestrogenic chemicals in body care cosmetics adversely*

affect breast cancer incidence in women? **Darbre, P. D., Harvey, P. W. and Parry, J. M.** 5, 2013, Journal of Applied Toxicology, Vol. 33, pp. 301-313.

406. *The effects of triclosan on puberty and thyroid hormones in male Wistar rats.* **Zorrilla, L. M., et al.** 1, 2009, Toxicological Sciences, Vol. 107, pp. 56-64.

407. *In vivo effects of bisphenol A in laboratory rodent studies.* **Richter, C. A., et al.** 2, 2007, Reproductive Toxicology, Vol. 24, pp. 199-224.

408. *Associations between socioeconomic status and environmental toxicant concentrations in adults in the USA: NHANES 2001–2010.* **Tyrrell, J., Melzer, D., et al.** 2013, Environment International, Vol. 59, pp. 328-335.

409. *The herbicide glyphosate is a potent inhibitor of 5-enolpyruvyl-shikimic acid-3-phosphate synthase.* **Steinrücken, H.C. and Amrhein, N.** 4, 1980, Biochem Biophys Res Commun., Vol. 94, pp. 1207-12.

410. *Impacts of genetically engineered crops on pesticide use in the U.S. -- the first sixteen years.* **Benbrook, C.M.** 2012, Environmental Sciences Europe, Vol. 24.

411. **EWG.** Roundup for Breakfast, Part 2: In New Tests, Weed Killer Found in All Kids' Cereals Sampled. [Online] 2018. https://www.ewg.org/news-insights/news-release/2018/10/roundup-breakfast-part-2-new-tests-weed-killer-found-all-kids.

412. **ABC Rural.** Glyphosate debate divides grain industry, sparks concern from livestock farmers. [Online] 1st November 2016. https://www.abc.net.au/news/rural/2016-11-01/glyphosate-herbicide-crops-grain-weeds-livestock-sheep-cattle/7982524.

413. **PIRG.** Glyphosate pesticide in beer and wine. [Online] 11th February 2019. https://pirg.org/resources/glyphosate-pesticide-in-beer-and-wine/.

414. *Pesticide Regulation amid the Influence of Industry.* **Boone, M.D., et al.** 10, 2014, Bioscience, Vol. 64, pp. 917–922.

415. *Differences in the carcinogenic evaluation of glyphosate between the International Agency for Research on Cancer (IARC) and the European Food Safety Authority (EFSA).* **Portier, C.J., et al.** 2016, Journal of Epidemiology & Community Health, Vol. 70, pp. 741-745.

416. **Sirinathsinghji, E. and Ho, M.W.** *Why Glyphosate Should Be Banned.* s.l. : Science in Society Archive, 2012.

417. *Determination of glyphosate and AMPA in blood and urine from humans: about 13 cases of acute intoxication.* **Zouaoui, K., et al.** 1-3, 2013, Forensic Sci Int., Vol. 226, pp. 20-5.

418. *Oxidative stress responses of rats exposed to Roundup and its active ingredient glyphosate.* **El-Shenawy, N.S.** 3, 2009, Environ Toxicol Pharmacol., Vol. 28, pp. 379-85.

419. *Cytotoxic and DNA-damaging properties of glyphosate and Roundup in human-derived buccal epithelial cells.* **Koller VJ, Fürhacker M, Nersesyan, A., et al.** 5, 2012, Arch Toxicol., Vol. 86, pp. 805-13.

420. *In vitro evaluation of genomic damage induced by glyphosate on human lymphocytes.* **Santovito, E., et al.** 2018, Environmental Science and Pollution Research, Vol. 25, pp. 34693–34700.

421. *Evaluation of DNA damage in an Ecuadorian population exposed to glyphosate.* **Paz-y-Miño, C., et al.** 2, 2007, Mutagenesis, Vol. 30.

422. *The toxicity of glyphosate alone and glyphosate-surfactant mixtures to western toad (Anaxyrus boreas) tadpoles.* **Vincent, K. and Davidson, C.** 12, 2015, Environ Toxicol Chem., Vol. 34, pp. 2791-5.

423. *Relative toxicity of the components of the original formulation of Roundup® to five North American anurans.* **Moore, L.J., et al.** 2012, Ecotoxicology and Environmental Safety, Vol. 78, pp. 128-133.

424. **Rueters, T.** Monsanto ordered to pay $289M US in California Roundup lawsuit over cancer claims. *CBC.* [Online] 10th August 2018.

https://www.cbc.ca/news/health/monsanto-payment-cancer-roundup-1.4781751.

425. **Levin, S. and Greenfield, P.** Monsanto ordered to pay $289m as jury rules weedkiller caused man's cancer. *The Guardian.* [Online] 2018 August 2018. https://www.theguardian.com/business/2018/aug/10/monsa nto-trial-cancer-dewayne-johnson-ruling.

426. **FSANZ.** Folic acid fortification. [Online] 19th January 2024. https://www.foodstandards.gov.au/consumer/food-fortification/folic-acid/folic-mandatory#:~:text=Australian%20and%20New%20Zealan d%20millers,for%20healthy%20growth%20and%20develo pment..

427. **FDA.** Food Additives Permitted for Direct Addition to Food for Human Consumption; Folic Acid. *Federal Register.* [Online] 15th April 2016. https://www.federalregister.gov/documents/2016/04/15/201 6-08792/food-additives-permitted-for-direct-addition-to-food-for-human-consumption-folic-acid#:~:text=Fortification%20with%20folic%20acid%20w as,effect%20on%20January%201%2C%201998..

428. *The Impact of Folic Acid Food Fortification on Global Incidence of Neural Tube Defects: Systematic Review, Meta-Analysis and Estimate of Preventable Cases.* **Brinkhof, M., et al.** Supp 1, 2015, International Journal of Epidemiology, Vol. 44, p. i143.

429. **Kapoor, D., et al.** Chapter 8 - Ligands for Targeted Drug Delivery and Applications. s.l. : Basic Fundamentals of Drug Delivery, 2019, pp. 307-342.

430. *Contribution of Dysregulated DNA Methylation to Autoimmunity.* **Funes, S.C., et al.** 21, 2021, Int J Mol Sci., Vol. 22.

431. *Homocysteine metabolism.* **Selhub, J.** 1999, Annu Rev Nutr., Vol. 19, pp. 217-46.

432. *Chemical Pathology of Homocysteine. IV. Excitotoxicity, Oxidative Stress, Endothelial Dysfunction,*

and Inflammation. **McCully, K.S.** 3, 2009, Annals of Clinical & Laboratory Science, Vol. 39, pp. 219-232.

433. *Homocysteine and atherothrombosis.* **Welch, G.N. and Loscalzo, J.** 15, 1998, N Engl J Med, Vol. 338, pp. 1042-50.

434. *Homocysteine impairs the nitric oxide synthase pathway: role of asymmetric dimethylarginine.* **Stühlinger, M.C., et al.** 21, s.l. : Circulation, 2001, Circulation, Vol. 104.

435. *The Dietary Effects of Methyl Donors on Asthma and Allergic Sensitization Is Influenced By the MTHFR C677T Polymorphism.* **Choi, Y.J., et al.** 2, Supp. AB104, 2016, Journal of Allergy and Clinical Immunology, Vol. 137.

436. *Association between MTHFR C677T/A1298C and susceptibility to autism spectrum disorders: a meta-analysis.* **Li, Y., et al.** 2020, BMC Pediatrics, Vol. 20.

437. *Folate and Inflammation – links between folate and features of inflammatory conditions.* **Jones, P., et al.** 2019, Journal of Nutrition & Intermediary Metabolism, Vol. 18.

438. *Homocysteine and MTHFR Mutations.* **Moll, S. and Varga, E.A.** 1, 2015, Circulation, Vol. 132.

439. *High risk of autoimmune diseases after COVID-19.* **Sharma, C. and Bayry, J.** 2023, at Rev Rheumatol, Vol. 19, pp. 399–400.

440. *Pre-existing conditions associated with post-acute sequelae of COVID-19.* **Jacobs, E.T., et al.** 2023, J Autoimmun, Vol. 135.

441. *Accelerated ageing is associated with increased COVID-19 severity and differences across ethnic groups may exist.* **Reeves, J., Kooner, J.S. and Zhang, W.** 2022, Front. Public Health, Vol. 10.

442. *Oxidative stress, aging, and diseases.* **Liguori, I., et al.** 2018, Clin Interv Aging, Vol. 13, pp. 757-772.

443. *Mold, Mycotoxins and a Dysregulated Immune System: A Combination of Concern?* **Kraft, S., Buchenauer, L. and Polte, T.** 22, 2021, Int J Mol Sci., Vol. 22.

444. *Co-infections: potentially lethal and unexplored in COVID-19.* **Cox, M. J., et al.** 1, 2021, The Lancet Microbe, Vol. 2, pp. e11-e12.

445. *Hydrogen and Methane-Based Breath Testing in Gastrointestinal Disorders: The North American Consensus.* **Rezaie, A., et al.** 5, 2017, The American Journal of Gastroenterology, Vol. 112, pp. 775-784.

446. *Candida: diagnosis and treatment.* **Pizzorno, J.** 6, 2014, Integrative Medicine: A Clinician's Journal, Vol. 13, pp. 8-12.

447. *The prevalence of small intestinal bacterial overgrowth in irritable bowel syndrome: an observation of the inconsistency between prevalence and testing methods.* **Pimentel, M.** 1, 2010, Gut Pathogens, Vol. 2, p. 3.

448. **Campbell, C. K. and Fyfe, J. A.** Candidiasis. [book auth.] T. M. Cox, & J. D. Firth (Eds.) D. A. Warrell. *Oxford Textbook of Medicine.* s.l. : Oxford University Press, 2011, pp. 1231-1235.

449. *Review article: lactose intolerance in clinical practice- -myths and realities.* **Lomer, M. C. E., Parkes, G. C. and Sanderson, J. D.** 2, 2014, Alimentary Pharmacology & Therapeutics, Vol. 39, pp. 110-121.

450. **Samaranayake, L. P., Fidel, P. L. and Naglik, J. R.** Fungal infections: Candidiasis. *Encyclopedia of Microbiology.* s.l. : Elsevier, 2009, pp. 223-233.

451. *Probiotics for the treatment of irritable bowel syndrome and small intestinal bacterial overgrowth.* **Pimentel, M. and et al.** 8, 2018, Journal of Clinical Gastroenterology, Vol. 52, pp. 702-712.

452. *Fermented foods and gastrointestinal health: A systematic review.* **Henshaw, E. and et al.** 5, 2020, Journal of Gastroenterology and Hepatology, Vol. 32, pp. 257-265.

453. *Association of a common variant of the endothelial nitric oxide synthase gene with cold-induced vasoconstriction and Raynaud's phenomenon.* **Maki-Petaja, K. M. and et al.** 8, 2007, Arteriosclerosis, Thrombosis, and Vascular Biology, Vol. 27, pp. 1840-1845.

454. *Nitric oxide synthase gene polymorphisms and Raynaud's phenomenon in systemic sclerosis.* **Miyamoto, Y. and et al.** 2, 2008, Rheumatology, Vol. 47, pp. 285-290.

455. *Raynaud's phenomenon.* **Wigley, F. M.** 14, 2002, The New England Journal of Medicine, Vol. 347, pp. 1001-1008.

456. —.**Block, J. A. and Sequeira, W.** 9273, 2001, The Lancet, Vol. 357, pp. 2042-2048.

457. *Clinical Effects of Regular Dry Sauna Bathing: A Systematic Review.* **Hussain, J. and Cohen, M.** 2018, Evidence-Based Complementary and Alternative Medicine.

458. *Sauna exposure leads to improved arterial compliance: Findings from a randomised controlled trial.* **Lee, E. and et al.** 2, 2018, European Journal of Preventive Cardiology, Vol. 25, pp. 130-138.

459. *Mechanisms and applications of the anti-inflammatory effects of photobiomodulation.* **Hamblin, M.R.** 3, 2017, AIMS Biophys., Vol. 4.

460. *Voluntary activation of the sympathetic nervous system and attenuation of the innate immune response in humans.* **Kox, M., et al.** 20, 2014, PNAS, Vol. 111, pp. 7379-7384.

461. *Cardiovascular and autonomic responses to physiological stressors before and after cold face test.* **Florian, J. P., et al.** 6, 2010, Physiological Measurement, Vol. 31, pp. 775–793.

462. *The effects of contrast water therapy on recovery and performance: A systematic review.* **Higgins, T. R. and McFarlane, N. T.** 10, 2014, Journal of Strength and Conditioning Research, Vol. 28, pp. 2731-2743.

463. *Alternating hot and cold water immersion for athlete recovery: A review.* **Cochrane, D. J.** 9, 2004, Journal of Sports Sciences, Vol. 22, pp. 819-827.

464. *Effects of cold water immersion on recovery: A review of protocols and temperatures.* **Cohen, A. J. and Pierrynowski, M. R.** 21, 2019, Journal of Sports Sciences, Vol. 37, pp. 2452-2462.

465. *Ice bath and contrast water therapy: A review of the evidence.* **Costello, J. T., Baker, P. R. and Cato, M.** 4,

2015, International Journal of Sports Medicine, Vol. 36, pp. 236-243.

466. *The fractal nature of nature: power laws, ecological complexity and biodiversity.* **Brown, J.H., et al.** 1421, s.l. : Philosophical Transactions of the Royal Society B, 2002, Vol. 357.

467. *The Fractal Nature of the Brain: EEG Data Suggests That the Brain Functions as a "Quantum Computer" in 5-8 Dimensions.* **Gardiner, J., Overall, R. and Marc, J.** 2, 2010, NeuroQuantology, Vol. 8, pp. 137-141.

468. *Does spending time outdoors reduce stress? A review of real-time stress response to outdoor environments.* **Kondo, M.C., Jacoby, S.F. and South, E.C.** s.l. : Health & Place, 2018, Vol. 51, pp. 136-150.

469. *Nature Exposure and Its Effects on Immune System Functioning: A Systematic Review.* **Anderson, L., Corazon, S.S. and Karlsson Stigsdotter, U.** 4, s.l. : Environmental Research and Public Health, 2021, Vol. 18.

470. *Viewing nature scenes positively affects recovery of autonomic function following acute-mental stress.* **Brown, D.K., Barton, J.L. and Gladwell, V.F.** 11, 2013, Environ Sci Technol., Vol. 37, pp. 5562-9.

471. **Chalmer, L.** How to Get the Most From Your Time in Nature. *Medium: Forge.* [Online] 27th July 2019. https://forge.medium.com/how-to-get-the-most-benefit-from-time-in-nature-8b58b44fd45e.

472. *Emotions, morbidity, and mortality: New perspectives from psychoneuroimmunology.* **Kiecolt-Glaser, J. K., et al.** 2002, Annual Review of Psychology, Vol. 53, pp. 83-107.

473. *Healthy places: Exploring the evidence.* **Frumkin, H.** 9, 2003, American Journal of Public Health, Vol. 93, pp. 1451-1456.

474. *Exercise-induced hormesis may help healthy aging.* **Ji, L.L., et al.** 1, 2010, Dose Response, Vol. 8, pp. 73-9.

475. *Mechanisms of exercise-induced mitochondrial biogenesis in skeletal muscle.* **Hood, D. A.** 3, 2009, Applied

Physiology, Nutrition, and Metabolism, Vol. 34, pp. 465-472.

476. *Maintenance of mitochondrial DNA integrity: repair and degradation.* **Kang, D. and Hamasaki, N.** 5, 2002, Current Genetics, Vol. 41, pp. 311-322.

477. *Free radicals in the physiological control of cell function.* **Dröge, W.** 1, 2002, Physiological Reviews, Vol. 82, pp. 47-95.

478. *Effect of TNF-alpha on PGC-1 expression in human muscle cells.* **Yu, M., et al.** 11, 2002, Diabetes, Vol. 51, pp. 3044-3049.

479. *Cytochrome c oxidase deficiency due to heme synthesis defect in a patient with lactic acidosis and motor neuropathy.* **Zong, H., Armoni, M., Harel, C., Karnieli, E., & Pessin, J. E.** 5, 2012, Journal of Clinical Investigation, Vol. 87, pp. 2053-2057.

480. *Autonomic adjustments to exercise in humans.* **Fisher, J. P., Young, C. N. and Fadel, P. J.** 2, 2015, Comprehensive Physiology, Vol. 5, pp. 475-512.

481. *Trends in oxidative aging theories.* **Muller, F. L., et al.** 4, 2007, Free Radical Biology and Medicine, Vol. 33, pp. 477-503.

482. *Exercise-induced oxidative stress: cellular mechanisms and impact on muscle force production.* **Powers, S. K. and Jackson, M. J.** 4, 2008, Physiological Reviews, Vol. 88, pp. 1243-1276.

483. *Antioxidant defenses: Mechanisms, methods, and results in oxidative stress.* **Jones, D. P. and et al.** 10, 2015, Nature Reviews Molecular Cell Biology, Vol. 16, pp. 671-683.

484. *Glutathione metabolism and its implications for health.* **Wu, G., et al.** 3, 2004, Journal of Nutrition, Vol. 134, pp. 489-492.

485. *Treadmill exercise training augments brain norepinephrine response to familiar and novel stress.* **Dishman, R. K., et al.** 3, 2006, Brain Research Bulletin, Vol. 42, pp. 399-406.

486. *Benefit from B-lymphocyte depletion using the anti-CD20 antibody rituximab in chronic fatigue syndrome: A double-blind and placebo-controlled study.* **Fluge, Ø., et al.** 2, 2016, PLOS ONE, Vol. 6.

487. *The anti-inflammatory effects of exercise: mechanisms and implications for the prevention and treatment of disease.* **Gleeson, M., et al.** 9, 2011, Nature Reviews Immunology, Vol. 11, pp. 607-615.

488. *Sympathetic skin response and its correlation with disease severity in rheumatoid arthritis.* **Pal, G. K., et al.** 4, 2013, Indian Journal of Physiology and Pharmacology, Vol. 57, pp. 339-347.

489. *Effect of high-intensity exercise on rheumatoid arthritis.* **Lemmey, A. B. and et al.** 3, 2009, Annals of the Rheumatic Diseases, Vol. 68, pp. 349-355.

490. *Exercise for osteoarthritis of the hip.* **Rausch Osthoff, A. K. and et al.** 2018, Cochrane Database of Systematic Reviews, Vol. 4.

491. *Autoimmune Basis for Postural Tachycardia Syndrome.* **Li, H. and et al.** 1, 2014, JAHA, Vol. 3.

492. *Hypertension as an autoimmune and inflammatory disease.* **Solak, Y. and et al.** 2016, Hypertension, Vol. 39, pp. 567–573.

493. **American Heart Association.** How high blood pressure is diagnosed. [Online] https://www.heart.org/en/health-topics/high-blood-pressure/the-facts-about-high-blood-pressure/how-high-blood-pressure-is-diagnosed.

494. *High-intensity interval exercise induces 24-h energy expenditure similar to traditional endurance exercise despite reduced time commitment.* **Skelly, L. E. and et al.** 7, 2014, Applied Physiology, Nutrition, and Metabolism, Vol. 39, pp. 845-848.

495. *Two minutes of sprint-interval exercise elicits 24-hr oxygen consumption similar to that of 30 min of continuous endurance exercise.* **Hazell, T.J., et al.** 4, 2012, Int J Sport Nutr Exerc Metab., Vol. 22, pp. 276-83.

496. **Huberman Lab.** Foundational Fitness Protocol. [Online] 2nd November 2022. https://www.hubermanlab.com/newsletter/foundational-fitness-protocol.

497. *Yoga improves mitochondrial health and reduces severity of autoimmune inflammatory arthritis: A randomized controlled trial.* **Gautam, S., et al.** 2021, Mitochondrion, Vol. 58, pp. 147-159.

498. *Therapeutic Effects of the Pilates Method in Patients with Multiple Sclerosis: A Systematic Review.* **Rodríguez-Fuentes, G., et al.** 2022, J. Clin. Med., Vol. 11.

499. *Maintenance of physical activity after Internet-based physical activity interventions in patients with rheumatoid arthritis.* **Hurkmans, E.J., et al.** 1, 2010, Rheumatology, Vol. 49, pp. 167–172.

500. *Supervised walking improves cardiorespiratory fitness, exercise tolerance, and fatigue in women with primary Sjögren's syndrome: a randomized-controlled trial.* **Tatiyama Miyamoto, S. and et al.** 2019, Clinical Trials, Vol. 39, pp. 227–238.

501. *Effects of a walking exercise programme on disease activity, sleep quality, and quality of life in systemic lupus erythematosus patients.* **Lin, M.C. and et al.** 6, 2023, International Journal of Nursing Practice, Vol. 29.

502. *The anti-inflammatory effects of exercise on autoimmune diseases: A 20-year systematic review.* **Luo, B., et al.** 3, 2024, Journal of Sport and Health Science, Vol. 13, pp. 353-367.

503. *Sleep deprivation in the rat: III. Total sleep deprivation.* **Everson, C.A., Bergmann, B.M. and Rechtschaffen, A.** 1, 1989, Sleep, Vol. 12, pp. 13-21.

504. *Short sleep duration is associated with reduced leptin, elevated ghrelin, and increased body mass index.* **Taheri, S., et al.** 3, 2004, PLoS Medicine, Vol. 1.

505. *Butyrate and propionate protect against diet-induced obesity and regulate gut hormones via free fatty acid*

receptor 3-independent mechanisms. **Lin, H. V., et al.** 4, 2012, PLOS ONE, Vol. 7.

506. *Role of gut microflora in the development of obesity and insulin resistance following high-fat diet feeding.* **Cani, P. D., et al.** 5, 2007, Pathologie Biologie, Vol. 56, pp. 305-309.

507. *Brief communication: Sleep curtailment in healthy young men is associated with decreased leptin levels, elevated ghrelin levels, and increased hunger and appetite.* **Spiegel, K., et al.** 11, 2004, Annals of Internal Medicine, Vol. 141, pp. 846-850.

508. *Sleep and metabolic function.* **Morselli, L., Guyon, A. and Spiegel, K.** 1, 2010, Pflügers Archiv - European Journal of Physiology, Vol. 459, pp. 139-150.

509. *Oxidative DNA damage in neurodegeneration.* **Evans, M. D. and Cooke, M. S.** 1, 2004, British Medical Bulletin, Vol. 71, pp. 187-201.

510. *Brown adipose tissue: Function and physiological significance.* **Cannon, B. and Nedergaard, J.** 1, 2004, Physiological Reviews, Vol. 84, pp. 277-359.

511. *The hunger genes: Pathways to obesity.* **van der Klaauw, A. A. and Farooqi, I. S.** 1, 2016, Cell, Vol. 161, pp. 119-132.

512. *Restlessness, impulsivity, and sleep in adults with attention-deficit/hyperactivity disorder (ADHD).* **Wynchank, D. and Bijlenga, D.** 3, 2018, Sleep Medicine Clinics, Vol. 13, pp. 235-240.

513. *Oxidative stress in university students during examinations.* **Sivonová, M., et al.** 3, 2004, Stress, Vol. 7, pp. 183-188.

514. *Sleep deprivation as a neurobiologic and physiologic stressor: Allostasis and allostatic load.* **McEwen, B. S.** 10 Supp 2, 2006, Metabolism: Clinical and Experimental, Vol. 55, pp. S20-S23.

515. **Sleep Health Foundation.** How much sleep do you really need? [Online] 2022. https://www.sleephealthfoundation.org.au/sleep-topics/how-much-sleep-do-you-really-

need#:~:text=Individuals%20vary%20in%20their%20sleep ,get%20away%20with%20less%20sleep..

516. *National Sleep Foundation's sleep time duration recommendations: Methodology and results summary.* **Hirshkowitz, M. and et al.** 1, 2015, Sleep Health, Vol. 1, pp. 40-43.

517. *Sleep duration and hypertension: Analysis of > 700,000 adults by age and sex.* **Grandner, M. A. and et al.** 5, 2010, Journal of Clinical Sleep Medicine, Vol. 6, pp. 497-504.

518. *Sleep deficiency and motor vehicle crash risk in the general population: A prospective cohort study.* **Czeisler, C. A. and et al.** 2015, BMC Medicine, Vol. 13, pp. 1-12.

519. **Walker, M. P.** *Why We Sleep: Unlocking the Power of Sleep and Dreams.* s.l. : Simon & Schuster, 2017.

520. *Development and validation of patient-reported outcome measures for sleep disturbance and sleep-related impairments.* **Buysse DJ, Yu L, Moul DE, Germain, A., et al.** 6, 2010, Sleep, Vol. 33, pp. 781-92.

521. **National Sleep Foundation.** 10 Tips for a Better Night's Sleep. [Online] https://www.thensf.org/sleep-tips/#:~:text=Make%20sure%20your%20bedroom%20is,de grees%20Fahrenheit%20helps%20promote%20sleep..

522. *The psychological benefits of moderate alcohol consumption: a review of the literature.* **Baum-Baicker, C.** 4, 1985, Drug Alcohol Depend., Vol. 15, pp. 305-22.

523. *The relationship between alcohol consumption and cortisol secretion in an aging cohort.* **Badrick, E., et al.** 3, 2008, J Clin Endocrinol Metab., Vol. 93, pp. 750-7.

524. *Nocturnal Hypoglycemia: Clinical Manifestations and Therapeutic Strategies Toward Prevention.* **Allen, K.V. and Frier, B.M.** 6, 2003, Endocrine Practice, Vol. 9, pp. 530-543.

525. *Collagen peptide supplementation before bedtime reduces sleep fragmentation and improves cognitive function in physically active males with sleep complaints.* **Thomas, C., et al.** 2024, Eur J Nutr, Vol. 64, pp. 323–335.

526. *Slow-wave sleep and the risk of Type 2 Diabetes in Humans.* **Tasali, E., et al.** 3, 2008, Proceedings of the National Academy of Sciences, Vol. 105.

527. *Sleep drives metabolic clearance from the adult brain.* **Xie, L. and et al.** 6156, 2013, Science, Vol. 342, pp. 373-377.

528. *Sleep and immune function.* **Besedovsky, L., Lange, T. Born, J.** 9, 2012, PLoS Biology, Vol. 10.

529. *Alcohol and the sleeping brain.* **Colrain, I.M., Nicholas, C.L. and Baker, F.C.** 2014, Handb Clin Neurol., Vol. 125, pp. 415-31.

530. *nterrelationship between Sleep and Exercise: A Systematic Review.* **Dolezal, B.A., et al.** 2017, Adv Prev Med. .

531. *The effect of exercise on sleep and fatigue in rheumatoid arthritis: a randomized controlled study.* **Durcan, L., Wilson, F. and Cunnane, G.** 10, 2014, J Rheumatol., Vol. 41, pp. 1966-73.

532. *The role of actigraphy in the study of sleep and circadian rhythms.* **Ancoli-Israel, S., et al.** 3, 2003, Sleep, Vol. 26, pp. 342-92.

533. *How sleep and mental disorders are related to complaints of daytime sleepiness.* **Ohayon, M.M., et al.** 22, 1997, Arch Intern Med., Vol. 157, pp. 2645-52.

534. *Circadian regulation of sleep in mammals: role of the suprachiasmatic nucleus.* **Mistlberger, R. E.** 3, 2005, Brain Research Reviews, Vol. 49, pp. 429-454.

535. *Role of Melatonin in the Regulation of Human Circadian Rhythms and Sleep.* **Cajochen, C., Krauchi, K. and Wirz-Justice, A.** 4, 2003, Journal of Neuroendocrinology, Vol. 15, pp. 432-437.

536. *Adverse metabolic and cardiovascular consequences of circadian misalignment.* **Scheer, F. A., et al.** 11, 2009, Proceedings of the National Academy of Sciences, Vol. 106, pp. 4453-4458.

537. *Physiology of growth hormone secretion during sleep.* **Van Cauter, E. and Plat, L.** Supp 3, 1996, Journal of Pediatric Endocrinology & Metabolism, Vol. 9, pp. 295-302.

538. *Growth hormone prevents the development of autoimmune diabetes.* **Villares, R., et al.** 48, 2013, PNAS, Vol. 110, pp. E4619-E4627.

539. *Neural mechanisms of hypnosis and meditation.* **Bendittis, G.** 4-6, 2015, Journal of Physiology-Paris, Vol. 109, pp. 152-164.

540. *Effects of perioperative clinical hypnosis on heart rate variability in patients undergoing oncologic surgery: secondary outcomes of a randomized controlled trial.* **Azam, M.A., et al.** 2014, Front. Pain Res., Vol. 5.

541. **REVERI.** [Online] https://www.reveri.com.

542. *The relationship between melatonin and cortisol rhythms: clinical implications of melatonin therapy.* **Zisapel, N., Tarrasch, R. and Laudon, M.** 3, 2005, Drug Development Research, Vol. 65, pp. 119-125.

543. *Effects of light on human circadian rhythms, sleep and mood.* **Blume, C., Garbazza, C. and Spitschan, M.** 3, 2019, Somnologie, Vol. 23, pp. 147-156.

544. *Adenosine, caffeine, and sleep-wake regulation: state of the science and perspectives.* **Reichert, C.F., Deboer, T. and Landolt, H.P.** 4, 2022, J Sleep Res., Vol. 31.

545. *Caffeine: Sleep and daytime sleepiness.* **Roehrs, T. and Roth, T.** 2, 2008, Sleep Medicine Reviews, Vol. 12, pp. 153-162.

546. *An update on the mechanisms of the psychostimulant effects of caffeine.* **Ferré, S.** 4, 2008, Journal of Neurochemistry, Vol. 105, pp. 1067-1079.

547. *Different responses of selected hormones to three types of exercise in young men.* **Stokes, K. A., et al.** 3, 2013, European Journal of Applied Physiology, Vol. 113, pp. 775-783.

548. *Creatine Activity as a Neuromodulator in the Central Nervous System.* **Meftahi, G.H., Hatef, B. and Pirzad**

Jahromi, G. 4, 2023, Arch Razi Inst., Vol. 78, pp. 1169-1175.

549. *GABA mechanisms and sleep.* **Gottesmann, C.** 2, 2002, Neuroscience, Vol. 111, pp. 231-9.

550. *Effects of vitamin and mineral supplementation on stress, mild psychiatric symptoms, and mood in non-clinical samples: A meta-analysis.* **Long, S. and Benton, D.** 2, 2013, Psychosomatic Medicine, Vol. 75, pp. 144-153.

551. *Magnesium and aging.* **Barbagallo, M. and Dominguez, L. J.** 7, 2010, Current Pharmaceutical Design, Vol. 16, pp. 832-839.

552. **Dean, C., Hickey, S. and Hickey, A.** *The magnesium miracle (Revised and Updated Edition).* s.l. : Ballantine Books, 2011.

553. *The effect of magnesium supplementation on primary insomnia in elderly: A double-blind placebo-controlled clinical trial.* **Abbasi, B., et al.** 12, 2012, Journal of Research in Medical Sciences, Vol. 17, pp. 1161-1169.

554. *Magnesium, inflammation, and obesity in chronic disease.* **Nielsen, F. H.** 6, 2010, Nutrition Reviews, Vol. 68, pp. 333-340.

555. *Subclinical magnesium deficiency: A principal driver of cardiovascular disease and a public health crisis.* **DiNicolantonio, J. J., O'Keefe, J. H. and Wilson, W.** 1, 2018, Open Heart, Vol. 5.

556. *Bioavailability of magnesium diglycinate vs magnesium oxide in patients with ileal resection.* **Schuette, S. A., Lashner, B. A. and Janghorbani, M.** 5, 1994, Journal of Parenteral and Enteral Nutrition, Vol. 18, pp. 430-435.

557. *Mg citrate found more bioavailable than other Mg preparations in a randomised, double-blind study.* **Walker, A. F., et al.** 3, 2004, Magnesium Research, Vol. 16, pp. 183-191.

558. *Brain-derived neurotrophic factor and its clinical implications.* **Liu, G., et al.** 4, 2016, Archives of Neurology, Vol. 62, pp. 575-584.

559. *Magnesium taurate effects on anxiety-like behavior and GABAergic/glutamatergic parameters in mice hippocampus under unpredictable chronic mild stress.* **Ferreira, A. G. K., et al.** 4, 2016, Magnesium Research, Vol. 29, pp. 160-167.

560. *Effect of transdermal magnesium chloride on serum and urinary magnesium levels in humans.* **Kass, L., et al.** 1, 2013, Journal of Evidence-Based Complementary & Alternative Medicine, Vol. 18, pp. 9-12.

561. *L-theanine, a natural constituent in tea, and its effect on mental state.* **Nobre, A. C., Rao, A. and Owen, G. N.** 1, 2008, Asia Pacific Journal of Clinical Nutrition, Vol. 17, pp. 167-168.

562. *The neuropharmacology of L-theanine (N-ethyl-L-glutamine): A possible neuroprotective and cognitive enhancing agent.* **Nathan, P. J., et al.** 2, 2006, Journal of Herbal Pharmacotherapy, Vol. 6, pp. 21-30.

563. *L-Theanine reduces psychological and physiological stress responses.* **Kimura, K., et al.** 1, 2007, Biological Psychology, Vol. 74, pp. 39-45.

564. *The effects of L-theanine (Suntheanine®) on objective sleep quality in boys with attention deficit hyperactivity disorder (ADHD): A randomized, double-blind, placebo-controlled clinical trial.* **Lyon, M. R., Kapoor, M. P. and Juneja, L. R.** 4, 2011, Alternative Medicine Review, Vol. 11, pp. 348-354.

565. *Effects of chronic l-theanine administration in patients with major depressive disorder: An open-label study.* **Hidese, S., et al.** 4, 2019, Acta Neuropsychiatrica, Vol. 31, pp. 169-177.

566. *Empirical treatment of insomnia.* **Orr, W. C., et al.** 3, 2008, General Hospital Psychiatry, Vol. 30, pp. 284-289.

567. *Translational value of rodent models in studying stress effects on sleep.* **Steenberg, L. M., et al.** 2020, Sleep Medicine Reviews, Vol. 51.

568. *The catechol-O-methyltransferase polymorphism: relations to the tonic-phasic dopamine hypothesis and*

neuropsychiatric phenotypes. **Bilder, R.M., et al.** 11, 2004, Neuropsychopharmacology, Vol. 29, pp. 1943-1961.

569. *Monoamine oxidase A gene polymorphism predicts adolescent outcome of attention-deficit/hyperactivity disorder.* **Li, J., et al.** 4, 2007, Am J Med Genet B Neuropsychiatr Genet, Vol. 144B, pp. 430-3.

570. *Val158Met polymorphisms of COMT gene and serum concentrations of catecholaminergic neurotransmitters of ADHD in Chinese children and adolescents.* **Xiong, Z., Yan, J. and Shi, S.** 49, 2021, Medicine, Vol. 100.

571. *Saffron (Crocus sativus) for depression: a systematic review of clinical studies and examination of underlying antidepressant mechanisms of action.* **Lopresti, A.L. and Drummond, P.D.** 6, 2014, Hum Psychopharmacol., Vol. 29, pp. 517-27.

572. *Effects of Saffron Extract on Sleep Quality: A Randomized Double-Blind Controlled Clinical Trial.* **Pachikian, B.D., et al.** 5, 2021, Nutrients, Vol. 13.

573. *The Emerging Role of Epigenetics in Autoimmune Thyroid Diseases.* **Wang, B., et al.** s.l. : Frontiers in Immunology, 2017, Vol. 8.

574. *A haplotype map of the human genome.* **The International HapMap Consortium.** 7063, 2005, Nature, Vol. 437, pp. 1299-1320.

575. **Klaassen, C. D. and Watkins, J. B.** *Casarett & Doull's Essentials of Toxicology (3rd ed.).* s.l. : McGraw-Hill Education, 2015.

576. *Homocysteine and MTHFR Mutations.* **Moll, S. and Varga, E.A.** 1, s.l. : Circulation, 2015, Vol. 231.

577. *MTHFR mutation: Another unifying etiology of chronic overlapping pain conditions.* **Visingardi, J., et al.** s.l. : Continence, 2023, Vol. 8. 101052.

578. *Association between variants of MTHFR genes and psychiatric disorders: A meta-analysis.* **Zhang, Y.X., et al.** s.l. : Front. Psychiatry, 2022, Vol. 13.

579. *Increased prevalence of methylenetetrahydrofolate reductase C677T variant in patients with inflammatory*

bowel disease, and its clinical implications. **Mahmud, N., et al.** s.l. : BMJ: Gut, 1999, Vol. 45, pp. 389-394.

580. *Methylenetetrahydrofolate reductase, MTHFR, polymorphisms and predisposition to different multifactorial disorders.* **Cristalli, C.P., et al.** s.l. : Genes & Genomics, 2017, Vol. 39.

581. *Cytochromes p450: roles in diseases.* **Pikuleva, I.A. and Waterman, M.R.** 24, s.l. : J Biol Chem. , 2013, Vol. 288.

582. *Effects and Mechanisms of Taurine as a Therapeutic Agent.* **Schaffer, S. and Won Kim, H.** 3, s.l. : Biomol Ther (Seoul), 2018, Vol. 26.

583. *Inherited disorders of bilirubin metabolism.* **Bosma, P.J.** 1, s.l. : Journal of Hepatology, 2003, Vol. 38.

584. *Glutathione in disease.* **Marvin, R. and Farook, J.** 4, s.l. : Clinical Nutrition and Metabolic Care, 2001, Vol. 1.

585. *Evidence for Accelerated Rates of Glutathione Utilization and Glutathione Depletion in Adolescents With Poorly Controlled Type 1 Diabetes.* **Darmaun, D., et al.** 1, s.l. : diabetes, 2005, Vol. 54.

586. *Impaired Glutathione Synthesis in Neurodegeneration.* **Aoyama, K. and Nakani, T.** 10, s.l. : International Journal of Molecular Sciences, 2013, Vol. 14.

587. *Contribution of dietary protein to sulfide production in the large intestine: an in vitro and a controlled feeding study in humans.* **Magee, E.A., et al.** 6, s.l. : Am J Clin Nutr, 2000, Vol. 72.

588. *Microbial pathways in colonic sulfur metabolism and links with health and disease.* **Carbonero, F., et al.** 3, s.l. : Front Physiol., 2012, Vol. 28.

589. *Sulfite sensitivity: significance in human health.* **Lester, M.R.** 14, s.l. : J Am Coll Nutr., Vol. 1995. 3.

590. *Hydrogen Sulfide in Skin Diseases: A Novel Mediator and Therapeutic Target.* **Xiao, Q., et al.** s.l. : Oxid Med Cell Longev., 2021. 6652086.

591. *Clinical aspects and diagnosis of sulfite intolerance. Apropos of 9 patients.* **Miltgen, J., et al.** 6, s.l. : Rev Pneumol Clin., 1996, Vol. 52.

592. **Sterer, N. and Rosenberg, M.** *Breath odors: origin, diagnosis, and management.* s.l. : Springer Science & Business Media, 2006.

593. *N-acetyltransferase and inflammation: Bridging an unexplored niche.* **Raghul Kannan, S. and Tamizhselvi, R.** s.l. : Gene, 2023, Vol. 887.

594. *Arylamine N-acetyltransferases: from drug metabolism and pharmacogenetics to drug discovery.* **Sim, E., Abuhammad, A. and Ryan, A.** 11, s.l. : Br J Pharmacol. , 2014, Vol. 171.

595. *Hypothesis: Hyperhomocysteinemia is an indicator of oxidant stress.* **Hoffman, M.** 6, 2011, Medical Hypotheses, Vol. 77, pp. 1088-1093.

596. *Thimerosal exposure and the role of sulfation chemistry and thiol availability in autism.* **Kern, J.K., et al.** 8, s.l. : Int J Environ Res Public Health, 2013, Vol. 10.

597. *The Link Between Hyperhomocysteinemia and Hypomethylation: Implications for Cardiovascular Disease.* **Barroso, M., Handy, D.E. and Castro, R.** 2017, Journal of Inborn Errors of Metabolism and Screening.

598. **VMNIS.** *Serum and red blood cell folate concentrations for assessing folate status in populations.* Geneva : WHO, 2012.

599. *Holotranscobalamin, a marker of vitamin B-12 status: analytical aspects and clinical utility.* **Nexo, E. and Hoffmann-Lücke, E.** 1, s.l. : Am J Clin Nutr, 2011, Am J Clin Nutr, Vol. 94, pp. 359S-365S.

600. *Methyl-Donor and Cofactor Nutrient Intakes in the First 2-3 Years and Global DNA Methylation at Age 4: A Prospective Cohort Study.* **Taylor, R.M., et al.** 3, 2018, Nutrients, Vol. 10.

601. *LINK BETWEEN METHYL NUTRIENTS AND THE DNA METHYLATION PROCESS IN THE COURSE OF SELECTED DISEASES IN ADULTS.* **Lobos, P. and**

Regulska-Ilow, B. 2, s.l. : Rocz Panstw Zakl Hig, 2021, Vol. 72.

602. *Folate and DNA Methylation.* **Ly, A., et al.** 2, s.l. : Antioxidants & Redox Signalling, 2012, Vol. 17.

603. *Folic Acid, Folinic Acid, 5 Methyl TetraHydroFolate Supplementation for Mutations That Affect Epigenesis through the Folate and One-Carbon Cycles.* **Menezo, Y., et al.** 2, s.l. : Biomolecules, 2022, Vol. 12.

604. *Cobalamin, the stomach, and aging.* **Carmel, R.** 4, s.l. : Am J Clin Nutr., 1997, Vol. 66.

605. *Betaine as a Functional Ingredient: Metabolism, Health-Promoting Attributes, Food Sources, Applications and Analysis Methods.* **Dobrijević, D., et al.** 12, s.l. : Molecules, 2023, Vol. 28.

606. *Folic acid: nutritional biochemistry, molecular biology, and role in disease processes.* **Lucock, M.** 1-2, s.l. : Mol Genet Metab, 2001, Vol. 71.

607. *Role of S-adenosyl-L-methionine in liver health and injury.* **Mato, J.M. and Lu, S.C.** 5, s.l. : Hepatology, 2007, Vol. 45.

608. *Cytochrome P450 Structure, Function and Clinical Significance: A Review.* **Manikandan, P. and Nagini, S.** 1, s.l. : Curr Drug Targets, 2018, Vol. 19.

609. *The current state of serum biomarkers of hepatotoxicity.* **Ozer, J., et al.** 3, 2008, Toxicology, Vol. 245, pp. 194-205.

610. *Drugs and the liver.* **R., Vaja and Rana, M.** 10, 2020, Anaesthesia and Intensive Care Medicine, Vol. 21, pp. 517–23.

611. *Hepatoprotective herbal drug, silymarin from experimental pharmacology to clinical medicine.* **Pradhan, S.C. and Girish, C.** 5, s.l. : Indian J Med Res., 2006, Vol. 124.

612. *Silymarin as a Natural Antioxidant: An Overview of the Current Evidence and Perspectives.* **Surai, P.F.** 1, s.l. : Antioxidants (Basel)., 2015, Vol. 4.

613. *Silymarin: a review of its clinical properties in the management of hepatic disorders.* **Wellington, K. and Jarvis, B.** 7, s.l. : BioDrugs, 2001, Vol. 15.

614. *A Randomized Controlled Clinical Trial in Healthy Older Adults to Determine Efficacy of Glycine and N-Acetylcysteine Supplementation on Glutathione Redox Status and Oxidative Damage.* **Lizzo, G., et al.** s.l. : Frontiers in Aging, 2022, Vol. 3.

615. *Supplementing Glycine and N-Acetylcysteine (GlyNAC) in Older Adults Improves Glutathione Deficiency, Oxidative Stress, Mitochondrial Dysfunction, Inflammation, Physical Function, and Aging Hallmarks: A Randomized Clinical Trial.* **Kumar, P., et al.** 1, s.l. : J Gerontol A Biol Sci Med Sci. , 2023, Vol. 78.

616. *Drug glucuronidation in humans.* **Miners, J.O. and Mackenzie, P.I.** 3, s.l. : Pharmacol Ther. , 1991, Vol. 51.

617. **NIH.** *UGT1A1 UDP glucuronosyltransferase family 1 member A1 [Homo sapiens (human).* 1st October 2024.

618. *Metabolic inactivation of estrogens in breast tissue by UDP-glucuronosyltransferase enzymes: an overview.* **Guillemette, C., Belanger, A. and Lepine, J.** 2004, Breast Cancer Research, Vol. 6.

619. **Vogel, V.G.** Epidemiology of Breast Cancer. *Science Direct: Estrogen Metabolism.* [Online] 2018. https://www.sciencedirect.com/topics/medicine-and-dentistry/estrogen-metabolism.

620. *The correlation between UDP-glucuronosyltransferase polymorphisms and environmental endocrine disruptors levels in polycystic ovary syndrome patients.* **Luo, Y., et al.** 11, 2020, Medicine, Vol. 99.

621. *Endometriosis and infertility: the hidden link between endometritis, hormonal imbalances and immune dysfunctions preventing implantation!* **Bouic, P.J.** 2, 2023, JBRA Assist Reprod., Vol. 27, pp. 144-146.

622. *Effect of calcium glucarate on beta-glucuronidase activity and glucarate content of certain vegetables and*

fruits. **Dwivedi, C., et al.** 2, 1990, Biochem Med Metab Biol., Vol. 43, pp. 83-92.

623. *Pharmacokinetic of berberine, the main constituent of Berberis vulgaris L.: A comprehensive review.* **Khoshandam, A., Imenshahidi, M. and Hosseinzadeh, H.** 11, s.l. : Phytotherapy Research, 2022, Vol. 36.

624. *Resveratrol Modulates Drug- and Carcinogen-Metabolizing Enzymes in a Healthy Volunteer Study.* **Chow, H.H.S., et al.** 9, 2010, Cancer Prevention Research, Vol. 3, pp. 1168–1175.

625. *Mechanisms Underlying Biological Effects of Cruciferous Glucosinolate-Derived Isothiocyanates/Indoles: A Focus on Metabolic Syndrome.* **Esteve, M.** 111, 2020, Front Nutr., Vol. 7.

626. *PharmGKB summary: pathways of acetaminophen metabolism at the therapeutic versus toxic doses.* **Mazaleuskaya, L.L., et al.** 8, 2015, Pharmacogenet Genomics, Vol. 25, pp. 416-26.

627. *Mitochondrial glutathione, a key survival antioxidant.* **Marí, M., et al.** 11, 2009, Antioxid Redox Signal., Vol. 11, pp. 2685-700.

628. *Glutathione dysregulation and the etiology and progression of human diseases.* **Ballatori, N., et al.** 3, 2009, Biol Chem., Vol. 390, pp. 191-214.

629. *Role of pyroglutamic acid in cumulus cells of women with polycystic ovary syndrome.* **Turathum, B., et al.** 12, 2022, J Assist Reprod Genet., Vol. 39, pp. 2737-2746.

630. *Glutathione is a key player in metal-induced oxidative stress defenses.* **Jozefczak, M., et al.** 3, 2012, Int J Mol Sci., Vol. 13, pp. 3145-3175.

631. *Regeneration of glutathione by α-lipoic acid via Nrf2/ARE signaling pathway alleviates cadmium-induced HepG2 cell toxicity.* **Zhang, J., et al.** 2017, Environ Toxicol Pharmacol., Vol. 51, pp. 30-37.

632. *Long-term supplementation with selenate and selenomethionine: Selenium and glutathione peroxidase (EC 1.11.1.9) in blood components of New Zealand women.*

Thomson, C.D., et al. 2, s.l. : British Journal of Nutrition, 1993, Vol. 69.

633. *Randomized controlled trial of oral glutathione supplementation on body stores of glutathione.* **Richie, J.P. Jr., et al.** 2, s.l. : Eur J Nutr., 2015, Vol. 54.

634. *The Role of Sulfotransferases in Liver Diseases.* **Xie, Y. and Xie, W.** 9, s.l. : Drug Metab Dispos., 2020, Vol. 48.

635. *Sulfite oxidizing enzymes.* **Feng, C., Tollin, G. and Enemark, J.H.** 5, s.l. : Biochim Biophys Acta., 2007, Vol. 1774.

636. *Impaired Sulfate Metabolism and Epigenetics: Is There a Link in Autism?* **Hartzell, S. and Seneff, S.** 10, 2012, Entropy, Vol. 14, pp. 1953-1977.

637. *The metabolism and significance of homocysteine in nutrition and health.* **Kumar A, Palfrey HA, Pathak R, Kadowitz PJ, Gettys, T.W. and Murthy, S.N.** 2017, Nutr Metab (Lond)., Vol. 14.

638. *Homeostatic impact of sulfite and hydrogen sulfide on cysteine catabolism.* **Kohl, J.B., Mellis, A.T. and Schwarz, G.** 4, 2018, British Journal of Pharmacology, Vol. 176, pp. 554-570.

639. *Discovery of human zinc deficiency: its impact on human health and disease.* **Prasad, A.S.** 2, 2013, Adv Nutr., Vol. 4, pp. 176-90.

640. *Identification of 8-Hydroxyquinoline Derivatives That Decrease Cystathionine Beta Synthase (CBS) Activity.* **Conan, P., et al.** 12, 2022, Int J Mol Sci., Vol. 23.

641. **Johnson, J.L.** *Handbook of Nuritionally Essential Mineral Elements.* s.l. : CRC Press, 1997.

642. **NIH.** Molybdenum: Fact Sheet for Health Professionals. [Online] 30th March 2021. https://ods.od.nih.gov/factsheets/Molybdenum-HealthProfessional/.

643. *Physiological actions of taurine.* **Huxtable, R.J.** 1, s.l. : Physiol Rev. , 1992, Vol. 72.

644. *Taurine Supplementation Lowers Blood Pressure and Improves Vascular Function in Prehypertension:*

Randomized, Double-Blind, Placebo-Controlled Study. **Sun, Q., et al.** 3, s.l. : Hypertension, 2016, Vol. 67.

645. *Discovery of human zinc deficiency: its impact on human health and disease.* **Prasad, A.S.** 2, s.l. : Adv Nutr., 2013, Vol. 4.

646. *Spotlight on protein N-terminal acetylation.* **Ree, R., Varland, S. and Arnesen, T.** 2018, Nature: Experimental & Molecular Medicine, Vol. 50, pp. 1–13.

647. *Melatonin Biosynthesis: The Structure of Serotonin N-Acetyltransferase at 2.5 Å Resolution Suggests a Catalytic Mechanism.* **Burgess Hickman, A., Klein, D.C. and Dyda, F.** 1, 1999, Molecular Cell, Vol. 3, pp. 23-32.

648. *Elevation of histamine levels in rat and mouse tissues by the deacetylation of administered N-acetylhistamine.* **Endo, Y.** 4, 1979, European Journal of Pharmacology, Vol. 60, pp. 299-305.

649. *L-Carnitine and acetyl-L-carnitine roles and neuroprotection in developing brain.* **Ferreira, G.C. and McKenna, M.C.** 6, s.l. : Neurochem Res., 2017, Vol. 42.

650. *Effects of acetyl-L-carnitine in Alzheimer's disease patients unresponsive to acetylcholinesterase inhibitors.* **Bianchetti, A., Rozzini, R. and Trabucchi, M.** 4, s.l. : Curr Med Res Opin., 2003, Vol. 19.

651. *Effects of glycine on metabolic syndrome components: a review.* **M., Imenshahidi and Hossenzadeh, H.** 5, s.l. : J Endocrinol Invest., 2022, Vol. 45.

652. *The effects of glycine on subjective daytime performance in partially sleep-restricted healthy volunteers.* **Bannai, M., et al.** 61, s.l. : Front Neurol., 2012, Vol. 3.

653. *Choline: critical role during fetal development and dietary requirements in adults.* **Zeisel, S.H.** s.l. : Annu Rev Nutr., 2006, Vol. 26.

654. *Copper at the Fungal Pathogen-Host Axis.* **García-Santamarina, S. and Thiele, D.J.** 31, s.l. : Copper at the Fungal Pathogen-Host Axis, 2019, Vol. 250.

655. *Integrative medicine and the role of modified citrus pectin/alginates in heavy metal chelation and detoxification-*

-five case reports. **Eliaz, I., Weil, E. and Wilk, B.** 6, s.l. : Forsch Komplementmed., 2007, Vol. 14.

656. *Anti-cancer activities of pH- or heat-modified pectin.* **Leclere, L., Cutsem, P.V. and Michiels, C.** 4, s.l. : Front Pharmacol., 2013, Vol. 8.

657. *Investigation of detoxification nature of activated carbons developed from Manilkara zapota and de oiled soya.* **Sujatha, S. and Sivarethinamohan, R.** Part 1, s.l. : Materials Today: Proceedings, 2020, Vol. 21, pp. 663-668.

658. *Inositol and Non-Alcoholic Fatty Liver Disease: A Systematic Review on Deficiencies and Supplementation.* **Pani, A., et al.** 11, s.l. : Nutrients, 2020, Vol. 12. 3379.

659. *D-chiro-inositol--its functional role in insulin action and its deficit in insulin resistance.* **Larner, J.** 4, s.l. : Int J Exp Diabetes Res ., Int J Exp Diabetes Res ., Vol. 31.

660. **NIH.** Magnesium Fact Sheet for Health Professionals. [Online] 2nd June 2022. https://ods.od.nih.gov/factsheets/Magnesium-HealthProfessional/.

661. *Probiotics: an overview of beneficial effects.* **Ouwehand, A.C., S., Salminen and Isolauri, E.** 1-4, s.l. : Antonie Van Leeuwenhoek, 2002, Vol. 82.

662. **National Institutes of Health.** What are the parts of the nervous system? [Online] 10th January 2018. https://www.nichd.nih.gov/health/topics/neuro/conditioninfo/parts.

663. *The role of the immune system in posttraumatic stress disorder.* **Katrinli, S., et al.** 2022, Nature: Transl Psychiatry, Vol. 12, p. 313.

664. *N-Acetylcysteine (NAC): Impact on Human Health.* **dos Santos Tenorio, M.C., et al.** 6, s.l. : Antioxidants, 2921, Vol. 10.

665. *Alpha-lipoic acid as a dietary supplement: molecular mechanisms and therapeutic potential.* **Shay, K.P., et al.** 10, s.l. : Biochim Biophys Acta., 2009, Antioxidants, Vol. 1790.

rmcontent.com/pod-product-compliance
ource LLC
v PA
`20426
v13B/426